Christine and Christian Schneider's story is exc[...] erful appeal not to ignore the hell that exists [...] the Christian faith is not an elevator to heaven [...] difference, here and now, for God and humani[...]

—Shane Claiborne, author, USA

This is a wonderful book—challenging, provocative and engaging. The reader will find themselves drawn in and deeply moved by its fast pace and powerful human stories.

—Kristin Jack, Asia Coordinator, Servants, NZ

I find the book to be outstanding. Absorbing. A very good read. Touching. Not at all sanctimonious. A guide for Christians of the 21st century.

—Dominik Klenk, Journalist and Prior of a Christian Ecumenical Community (OJC) in Reichelsheim, Germany

This is not simply a book I have read and recommend. These are people that I know and a ministry that I have seen grow before my very eyes. It is the challenging story of doing urban mission among poor street young people in the challenging city of Metro Manila. This is story of incarnational love and concern. It is a story of hope. Its heartbeat may even move you.

—Charles Ringma, Research Professor Asian Theological Seminary, Manila; Emeritus Professor Regent College, Vancouver

Christine and Christian Schneider lived in the slums of Manila for ten years. Each day they shared the poverty of the poorest of the poor in order to give them back their dignity—and renewed hope.

—Lise Favre, former Swiss Ambassador to the Philippines

The Schneiders depict razen criminals and petty scoundrels, murderers, prostitutes, and junkies as their—yes!—amiable neighbors, who are *liebenswürdig*—worthy of God's love.

—Andreas Malessa, Author, Radio, and Television Journalist, Germany

Though this book is set amongst the rubble of Manila's slums, it is anything but hopeless. A truly inspiring story of redemption from the ground up—a grass-roots transformation that was sparked by an ordinary family who were willing to move into one of the most impoverished neighborhoods in the world. Read this book and prepare to be challenged.

—Craig Greenfield, International Coordinator of Servants, author of *The Urban Halo*, co-author of *Living Mission*, activist and missionary amongst the urban poor, Canada

Many of us hear the call. The still small voice that calls us to care. To care for all people—especially the poor—whom very few really care for. But unlike most of us, Chris and Christine Schneider listened to the call. They took the risk to act on the word they heard in their heart. They flew from the hermetically-sealed squeaky-clean safety and comfort of Switzerland into the full-on in-your-face poverty and violence on the city streets of the Philippines. And there, living among troubled people in the "rubble" of their lives, Chris and Christine prayed and plotted "redemption." *Rubble and Redemption* is their amazing story. It is a story for all of us who hope against hope. It is a story for all of us who want be the change we want to see in the world. And it is a story for all of us who have heard the call, to be reminded that now is the time for us to act on our call.

—Dave Andrews, author and activist, Australia

I can smell them as I read—the foul odors of the slums of Manila. Nothing is left out or glossed over. Above all, however, hope shines brightly, giving us the courage never to give up, neither on ourselves or others.

—Ruedi Josuran, coach and moderator, Switzerland

RUBBLE & REDEMPTION

Finding life in the slums of Manila

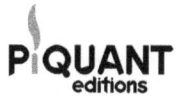

Christian and Christine Schneider
translated from German by Dagmar Grimm

PIQUANT editions

servants   Réseau Michée / Rede Miquéias / Red Miqueas / Micah Network   Onesimo

Copyright © Christian and Christine Schneider, 2012
The moral right of Christian and Christine Schneider to be identified as the authors of this work has been asserted in accordance with the Copyright, Designs and Patents Act of 1988.

Translated into English by Dagmar Grimm
First published in English by PIQUANT, 2012: Piquant Editions is an imprint of PIQUANT:
PO Box 83, Carlisle, CA3 9GR, UK
www.piquanteditions.com
ISBN 978-1-903689-78-3

Originally published in German as *Himmel und Strassenstaub: Unser Leben als Familie in den Slums von Manila* (Giessen: Brunnen, 2011)

British Library Cataloguing in Publication Data

Schneider, Christian.
  Rubble and redemption : finding life in the slums of
Manila.
  1. Schneider, Christian. 2. Schneider, Christine. 3. Church
work with the poor--Philippines--Manila. 4. Poor--
Medical care--Philippines--Manila.
  I. Title II. Schneider, Christine.
  362.1'086942'0959916-dc23

ISBN-13: 9781903689783

All Rights Reserved.
No part of this publication may be reproduced, stored in a retrieval system, or transmitted in any form or by any means, electronic, mechanical, photocopying, recording, or otherwise, without the prior permission of both the copyright owner and the publisher or a licence permitting restricted copying. In the UK such licences are issued by the Copyright Licensing Agency Ltd. www.cla.co.uk

Names of people may have been changed for the sake of anonymity.

Photo Credits:
p. 218 ©Friedel Ammann—Basel
All others by the authors

Cover design by Daniel Böhm
Book design by projectluz.com

www.piquanteditions.com
www.servantsasia.org
www.micahnetwork.org
www.onesimo.ch

For Rose Pecio-Salve,
Who lives with her family in the slums of Manila by choice and represents all
our Filipino friends similarly engaged in the Philippines.

and

For Ernst "Aschi" Bucher-Läng,
Who lives with his family in a remote Alpine valley
and represents all our friends in the affluent West who are not indifferent to
the poor in this world.

Contents

About this Book 1
Welcome to Bagong Silang 3
Childhood in Basel 7
England and Manila 11
Blessed are those who receive 13
Noriel, the Teenager 15
Ana and Rodelio 16
Jonar's Death 17
My Little Clinic 20
Mrs. Mercy 23
Jolli 25
Death in the Chapel 27
Nardo, the Resistance Fighter 29
Mata, the "Bodyguard" 32
Ruth, the Doctor 34
James, the Trades Union Steward 37
Imprinted Images 39
Snake Island 41
The Left Curve 43
Reymond, the Teenager 46
Moving to Bagong Barrio 48
The Freedom of a Motorcyclist 50
The War 52
Nick, the Witness 54
Moving to Potrero 57
Christmas Stories 59
Ate Donita, the Supplicant 61
Reunion with Christine 64
The Corpses Will Be Buried Later 69
Paulo 72
Rico, the Resolute 76
Faith for Cash 78
Navotas 81
Two Angels and a Motorcycle 84
Tired 86
Katja, the Temporary Missionary 88
The Fresh Breeze 91
If She Survives 93
More Swiss, Less Slum 96
Interim Balance 98

Romance is Sometimes Not Enough	100
A Challenging Entry into a Dynamic Life	103
A Difficult Birth	105
Letters from Manila	108
Beginnings in the NIA Slum	112
Letters from Manila	114
At Home in NIA	116
Letter from Manila	117
The Mountain of Rubbish	117
Letter from Manila	119
Culture Shock	119
The Payatas Gang	120
Rain Season	122
Doubly Pregnant	123
Letter from Manila	124
The Vision "Onesimo"	125
Make Way for Camp Rock	126
"Your Shack is on Fire!"	127
Noteworthy Contrasts	130
Sometimes Heaven Helps …	131
… and Sometimes a Revolver	133
A Therapeutic Communal Organization	136
Letter from Manila	138
Beginning of the Communal Organization	139
Learning to Live Together	141
Two Busses, One Nightmare	143
Letter from Manila	144
Paths to the World of Work	145
Letters from Manila	147
The Vultures of Payatas	148
Letter from Manila	151
An Easter Experience	152
Workcamp and the Everyday	153
September Days	156
"I didn't think that he would hurt me"	160
Tropical Fever	163
Letter from Manila	164
Moving to Philcoa	165
Summer Camps and "Women's Work"	167
The Community of Girls	169
Letter from Manila	170
Our Neighbors, the Billionaires	170

Trust is Priceless	173
Letters from Manila	174
Payatas in the World News	176
Flowing (Waste) Water	178
Controversy about Corpses	179
Everything that we do here is sensitive . . .	180
Three Filipinos in Switzerland	182
September 11th	183
Letter from Manila	183
A Bridge between Rich and Poor	186
Letters from Manila	188
Melancholy Christmas	189
Letter from Manila	191
Life Goes On	194
. . . and what became of them	196
Epilogue	207
Acknowledgements	209
More books from Servants Authors	210
Contact Addresses	210

About this Book

On a hot summer day in 1988, with my heart pounding and no idea what to expect, I moved into the Philippine Bagong Silang. This slum/resettlement area in Manila became my first home on my journey with the poor. For four years, I lived in the slums as a bachelor and subsequently for nine years with my family. While there, I came into contact with misery, poverty, beauty, and a love of life at very close range. Above all, I met people whose hospitality, will to survive, and faith transformed me. These encounters are central to my story.

We, as a family, returned to Switzerland over seven years ago. Once again we live in an affluent society, with its compulsion to consume and its emphasis on productivity, and with the extreme stress which one experiences in order to live comfortably, pleasurably, and securely.

This book is my attempt to hold fast cherished memories before they fade in the unavoidable crush of the daily activities of our Western lives. While sifting through letters and diary entries, I realized that many of my recollections are only snapshots; in many cases, I don't know how the stories of these people evolved after my departure.

Even though we again live in Switzerland, a part of us remained in the slums. Most probably we'll never lose the perspective of the "urban poor," and that's good. Regular trips to Manila temper my "homesickness." There I encounter the people of that time and the memories are reawakened. Many of these reunions are heartening; others make me feel sad.

My close friends and co-travelers in the story gave me the permission to use their real names. The names of others have been changed to protect their privacy.

—Christian Schneider

Welcome to Bagong Silang

June 9, 1988. Seemingly endless rows of the most remarkable dwellings cluster together on a sloping terrain seared by the harsh tropical sun. The blistering heat of summer shimmers above thousands of corrugated tin roofs. The "better" houses are built of crude cement bricks or thin plywood. And the further we distance ourselves from the main street, the more makeshift the dwellings become.

Rob Ewing, a slim, blond Australian, whose light blue eyes are alight with the resolve of a pioneer, leads me further and deeper into this shantytown of the displaced. We walk past derelict shacks, some looking like colorful collages made of old rice sacks, plastic sheeting, and cardboard boxes. I'm struck by how much they resemble refugees' camps in a war zone, and a feeling of apprehension overwhelms me. For these people, as a white man, I am rich, above all. An alien being. Nonetheless, I follow my guide to the lodgings of a family where I am to live for the next several months.

Bagong Silang lies a good hour's drive from the center of Manila. Rob estimates that 140,000 people live here, not a single one by choice. They've been deported to this place because the illegal squatters' slums where they lived before were razed to make way for new communities.

"*Bagong Silang* means new life," Rob explains. "But many people get sick here, and every day some die because of the polluted water or from starvation." Rob Ewing, with his wife, Lorraine, and his little daughter, has already been living in this area for three years. A small congregation of 60 to 80 believers, The Living Spring Christian Fellowship, has formed around this Australian family working with Servants (www.servantsasia.org). They have also established a small kindergarten and a soup and rice kitchen, where emaciated mothers bring their malnourished children once a day. Considering the misery of the masses, this little bit of aid strikes me as a bad joke. The people of Bagong Silang have been promised start-up help, but a few square yards of barren land and a ceramic toilet bowl are all the government agents ever provide for these evacuees to begin their new life.

Water towers, fifteen feet high and evenly dispersed, loom over the parched land. The tanks are empty and are rusting away. So as not to die of thirst, the residents fetch water from holes that they have dug themselves, but the water is befouled by the countless toilet pits close by where people relieve themselves.

One walks slowly in the settlement, with legs spread wide. The paths between the houses are narrow, with a drainage ditch in the middle covered with planks that the involuntary settlers often divert from their intended use to become building materials instead.

We arrive at the house of Nanay (Mother) and Tatay (Father) Opiasa. Quickly a small crowd gathers. Several little children take my hands without asking and squeeze them. Curiously and with affection, they pinch my arms with their dirty little fingers. A hefty woman, well over fifty, materializes in front of me. Yelling and thrashing her arms, she chases the children away. Then she looks me in the eye. I take her hand, bow my head, and guide the back of her hand to my forehead. I am asking for her blessing, a gracious, time-honored gesture that indicates warmth and respect for older people in this country.

"So this is Chris from Switzerland," she says in broken English. "Don't worry, Rob, we'll take good care of him." I don't doubt it for a second. "Chris, you are now my son . . . and just so you know, I am your mother." She laughs hoarsely and discreetly throws her cigarette stub away. "Mother," in this case, probably means "boss."

Before I can say anything, she pulls me into the cool shade of her *Sala,* the living room. With approximately two hundred seventy square feet, the room constitutes the floor plan of the house. It is the bedroom, dining room, kitchen—everything at once. The floor consists of stamped earth, the walls of raw cement brick. Above the much-too-low wood-plank ceiling, an upper room has been constructed with thin plywood and covered with corrugated tin. Openings draped with rice sacks serve as a kind of window. This will be my home for several months.

I notice that there is neither a family altar with candles and food offerings nor statues of saints in the shack. This suggests that the parents have turned away from the hybrid Philippine Catholicism that incorporates Filipino and Roman traditions. Mother Nanay Opiasa places wonderful ice-cold water on the rickety wooden table. The family owns a refrigerator and an old television. These two treasures have been provided by the savings of Nardo, the oldest son of the six Opiasa children. For six long years, he worked at construction sites in the Saudi Arabian desert. Nothing remains of his savings except for the television and this very refrigerator, which now continually produces ice, except when the power fails. This happens quite often and lasts for days and sometimes weeks—they call these surprises "blackouts." But when the power is on, Tatay Opiasa packs the ice in plastic and sells it to the neighbors for a few *centavos* apiece. A profitable sideline, it seems.

Nardo speaks the best English in the family and will be my language Helper. He and his wife, Jovelyn, and their six-month old baby live and sleep on the only wooden bed-like piece of furniture sequestered by a curtain in the *Sala*. Berna, the yet unmarried adult daughter, and the two teenage sons, Dario and Noriel, roll out their woven mats—*banig*—wherever they find room to sleep. The other two children have already moved out and have families of their own; in their stead, two dogs and five pigeons now reside under the same roof. The latter are the hobby of Noriel, the youngest. An old sofa is placed against the outer wall of the house, protected by a plastic awning; the parents sleep there.

Nanay Opiasa chats animatedly with Rob. The Filipinos' language appeals to me, but I can hardly imagine how I will be able to master these strange and complicated sounds one day. At the same time, this is the main goal of my first year here: To learn the language and customs of these people by living with them.

Presumably Rob and Nanay are discussing the expenses of the Opiasa family, as well they should. Their current living situation is to be improved in order to become bearable for me. Rob has given them money so that they can put a door that closes on the toilet room. The toilet is a ceramic siphon contraption, and one has to squat to do one's business. The septic tank under the shack appears to be sealed with a concrete cover, and a bucket full of water with an empty can that serves as a shower completes the space. It's not exactly the Grand Hotel, but I'll manage.

While we're under the tin roof using some plywood to construct a small place to sleep that should shield me from prying eyes, Rob's wife, Lorraine, arrives. She is tall and slender, with red hair and a light complexioned, freckled face, which distinguishes her markedly from the Filipino women. "Are you interested in coming with me on a couple of visits to the sick?" she asks with a smile. She knows that I'm a state-qualified nurse.

A short time later I'm holding a wrinkled bundle with large dark eyes in my hands. It is the severely undernourished newborn of a teenager, currently being cared for by her young grandmother. Little Jessabel has a mouth and jaw deformity which apparently hinders her in taking in sufficient amounts of food. Without professional help, the child has no chance of survival.

"She must go to the hospital immediately," I hear myself say, realizing at the same moment, however, how stupid this advice is. As if the family had the money for a long hospital stay! In state-run hospitals, relatives are required to pay for care and meals themselves, as well as for transportation and medication which are as expensive here as in the wealthy West. Lorraine indicates to me that the grandmother regularly avails herself of milk powder from the nutrition program of Servants.

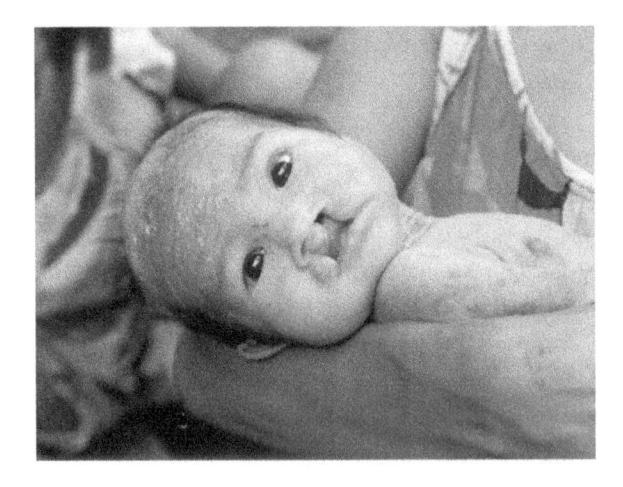

Jessabel* 1988:
Will she survive?
See page 195.

So what can we do? We lay our hands on these sad people with their beautiful smiles and wrap our arms around them and pray—to stave off despair and bring on recovery.

We step outside and stretch our limbs; many of the huts are too low for Caucasians. "Would you like to look in on another sick girl, just next door?" Lorraine asks. In Bagong Silang, the distance between one sick girl and the next is not very far.

"Mother will be back soon," a couple of children explain, poking their heads out of an opening in the wall of the house. "She has gone to an expensive doctor with our sister; she had another one of her attacks."

"Back soon," I've already learned, can mean anything; waiting seems to be a part of life here. The people have nothing but time, which they have in abundance. We sit down on improvised stools made of rubber tires and bamboo. It's already late afternoon; if it weren't for the stinging assaults of the mosquitoes, I could enjoy the fresh evening breeze. Near the equator, night falls suddenly after a brief but colorful twilight, and for most people this is the most pleasant time of the day. Young and old come out of their shacks and chat and play and argue and laugh.

All of a sudden, a small group of people approaches. Leading the way, a young woman comes toward us, her face the visage of naked despair. She carries her daughter in her arms; because of an epileptic attack, the six-year-old girl has suffocated on the way. Children of all ages and also adults crowd around

---

* Names of people may have been changed for the sake of anonymity.

the little corpse, many touching the still soft body one last time. They pray and weep loudly. We weep and pray, too.

Disconcerted, we walk home, each lost in our own thoughts. I suspect that in this place no one will really bother about the exact cause of death of the girl. The blaring of old radio and television amplifiers turned up too loud and the clamor of countless voices dominate the nighttime atmosphere of the wretched slum. "Welcome to Bagong Silang," Rob suddenly says, dryly. He knows what's on my mind and answers my unstated questions. "It's remarkable that the suffering and death of these little ones sometimes lead people to turn to God in their despair, to seek comfort and perhaps even the strength to orient their lives in a new direction."

Later that evening, I'm sitting under my mosquito net and sweating. Below my sleeping corner there's a huge racket. About forty children and young people from the neighborhood are crowded around the Opiasas' television. Heads poke through the open doors and the two window openings and loudly shout out comments about the current championship basketball game. For them this was a normal day.

Despite fatigue and unfamiliar sleeping quarters, I feel certain that I've arrived where another has led me, without my having sought it out. How odd—and how comforting. Slipping into an old habit, I read a few sentences in the Bible before falling asleep. They serve me well. My calmness strikes me as incongruous. It isn't even death that preoccupies me; as a nurse and caregiver to the terminally ill, I have often been confronted with dying adults. What bothers me is the senselessness of *this* death of *this* girl, while other parts of the same world drown in excess. *That* is incongruous, and not the calm within me.

I hope that I have the capacity to maintain my calm as long as I am here. I adjust as comfortably as I can to my narrow bed. At least it won't depend on that. I learned as a child how to get along with little space and even less privacy.

Childhood in Basel

As a young boy, I shared a small room with my two older brothers. Our eight family members lived in a four-room apartment in public housing on the outskirts of the city of Basel. Space to play outdoors was almost boundless. There was a gravel pit just a few minutes away by foot on French soil, which we were forbidden to trespass, beside wide, undeveloped fields with wild hedgerows and overgrown trenches that remained from the world wars. The open spaces were playing fields full of adventure. Here we smoked our first cigarettes, practiced with our bows and arrows and our sling shots, and resorted to violent brawling with other children who wanted to take over our space.

In contrast, attending school was an annoying matter of secondary importance. Far more important than our lessons, it seemed to me, was to be the strongest on the playground. Outside, there was adventure; inside, there was only boredom. Comments such as "conduct unsatisfactory" and "provisionally advanced" appeared on my report cards.

Every Wednesday, however, I took part in a "Children's Hour." We heard stories from the Bible, often with the message that God loves me and sent his son, Jesus, into the world especially for me so that he could make my heart pure. This impressed me deeply, since I often did battle with my feelings of guilt. One day I stayed behind with the Children's Hour mentor and responded to her invitation "to allow Jesus to enter my heart" with a prayer. I was seven-years-old and from that day forward I knew deep within me there was a God whom I could not ignore and who would never abandon me.

Nevertheless, "Jesus in my heart" had hardly any effect on my usual leisure activities. These included vandalism and shoplifting. I was never caught; if the pilfered goods could not be consumed immediately without a trace, I would toss them away as a precaution. In the evenings, I enjoyed throwing stones and shattering the electric street lamps. Once, an older boy chose to exclude me and play with other boys, which hurt my feelings so deeply that I started a fire in a playhouse that he had built himself, and ran away. As I saw the column of smoke and heard the fire engines from a distance, however, I didn't feel proud of myself. . . .

A turning point occurred with my entry into the Young Man's Christian Association (CVJM). I was eleven-years-old, and there was hardly a Saturday afternoon that I would not go there. The leaders were interested in my life; they brought me in closer contact with the city and the surrounding hills and forests, and I considered their fatherly friendship as a new and unfamiliar blessing. They told us stories from the Bible, and besides the novels by Karl May and comic books, I began to read the Bible.

These so-called "Jungschar," an Outdoor Children's Club, became the highpoints of my life. I formed friendships with young boys who came from "good backgrounds," and who were going to college-prep high schools (*Gymnasia*). In the CVJM there didn't seem to be any class differences. Most important, I began to commune with God more intensively. I accepted the ability to leave my kleptomania behind as significant proof that my prayers had been heard. In previous years I had often cried myself to sleep, overcome with guilt because I couldn't stop stealing.

After I finished school, I began vocational training as an engineering draftsman. In addition, I had two passions: Mountain climbing and CVJM.

I had plenty of reasons to flee into the mountains and to the CVJM: One of my older brothers had slipped completely into the drug scene, and the other one attempted suicide several times. Fortunately, at least my three younger siblings had found stability in work with young people in the CVJM. For me, there was nothing more compelling than to experience the way in which other people found their way to God, whom I had learned to know myself, and how they gained strength and joy in life by doing so. That's what I wanted to live for, and so I accepted ever greater responsibility in the Christian youth ministry.

My parents separated, much too late in my opinion, since they often seemed to be involved in major confrontations. At age 18, I rented a room, concluded my studies as a draftsman, and decided to train for a second vocation as a qualified nurse. It was a difficult year financially, but again and again I discovered envelopes with money in my mailbox, sent by people whom I had never told about my limited funds, and who weren't particularly close to me.

Three years of practical experience in a hospital setting made it abundantly clear to me that being a medical nurse was my "dream job." Even the communal life in two residential communities was, for me, a great enrichment. In my free time, I trained as a youth leader in sports such as hiking, skiing, and mountain climbing.

In 1980, my friends at CVJM persuaded me to establish a new children's ministry in Riehen, a wealthy suburb of Basel. With a younger friend I moved to the other side of the city and began my own youth group. In addition, we rented an old ten-room villa with a large garden which, in a very short time, became populated by an illustrious group. My frail grandfather; my mother, who had divorced my father in the meantime; my alcoholic uncle; and from time to time, my brother Roland, who had recently been released from drug rehab. Girlfriends from the drug scene, people adrift, and single colleagues from the youth group also lived with us. My mother took on most of the work of the residential community, insisting again and again that it made her happy. She had an unwavering belief in God, an unheard of empathy for the weak, and an enormous vitality that impressed me.

My life, which consisted of the hospital, children's ministry, residential community, and adventures in the mountains (the latter experienced most of the time with my best friend, Urs Mayer), came to a turning point when two theology students moved into our community. Ralf Dörpfeld and Volker Heitz took me to the streets and squares of Basel, where they preached with theater and song and where they engaged in conversations with passersby. For me this was a trial by fire—to openly declare myself as a Christian in my home town. At the same time, it gave my faith a new impetus. I assisted with the founding of a new Free Church, which grew very quickly and was later known as the Evangelical Community Basel.

My brother Erich, who is four years younger than I and also active in the Young Men's Christian Association, fell in love during this time with a young woman named Christine Tanner. She, however, did not reciprocate his feelings. The reasons why were unclear to me since he was a good looking, sporty type. Erich had a significant artistic talent, which led him to complete his studies at the School of Applied Arts in Basel. I was quite proud of my brother; in contrast, I perceived Christine as a cool and unapproachable beauty.

After four years my friends advised me to give up my profession and to apply my strengths to Christian endeavors full time. A training program in community building in England was recommended, after which I could study theology and cross-culture communication at a well known "Mission College." But that didn't appeal to me. First of all, I loved my work as a nurse and secondly, I didn't want to earn money as a "professional Christian." Therefore I applied to three educational institutions that trained caregivers as teachers, with vocational guidance and instruction in the field. To my surprise, I was accepted by all three schools. At the same time, an ulcer was discovered in my intestine. I didn't take it very seriously although my doctor warned me that the condition was potentially dangerous and that I should take my foot off the gas pedal a bit.

I drew up a balance sheet: I was twenty-seven-years-old; my colleagues in the Young Men's Christian Association children's ministry in Riehen, which had grown from eighteen to eighty children, were competent; the group had the ongoing support of older Christians in town; the lease on our residential villa would expire in a year. So I allowed myself to be convinced and moved to England in 1984 with the blessings of the congregation, the residential community, and the CVJM.

England and Manila

England was a new world. In my first year there, I fell into the midst of a spiritual uprising in an evangelical Free Church that called itself the "Ichthus" movement. The people practiced New Testament gifts such as healing the sick or speaking in tongues. Modern religious services, including a great deal of music and absorbing Bible readings with everyday practical interpretations, were conducted in school auditoriums. I took part in the founding of small branch communities in Southeast London, avidly traversing the streets between the graffiti-covered towers of the dark public housing apartments, attempting conversations with the residents.

During the next two years I took a diploma course at the All Nations Christian College (ANCC) not far from Cambridge. Since the academic year in England consists of three ten-week semesters, twenty weeks remained in which I could work in Switzerland as a nurse in order to finance my studies. In this way I was also able to remain in contact with my friends and family in Basel.

In addition to theology, I was particularly inspired in my studies by subjects concerning other religions and cultures. Half of the instructors came from the Third World. They often raised questions without giving answers. This broadened my horizon and my thought process, especially regarding questions of faith.

A practicum was required in the second year. I was impressed by the lectures about urban missions, and heard of a small, dauntless group from New Zealand, the Servants, who lived with the poor in the slums of Manila in the most abject circumstances. I came across the book *Companion to the Poor* by Viv Grigg. In the book, he describes his months in the slums and challenges Christians to pledge their lives to solidarity with the poor.

At the same time I received an invitation to join a well known North American missionary organization, whose missionaries work among neglected children and young people in traditional ways. I flew to Manila and determined to compare two basically different missionary concepts.

The North American missionary group was an impressive discovery: Most of the forty foreign colleagues lived in complete American luxury in the heavily guarded wealthy areas of the city. The work in the streets, in the prisons, and nursing homes was performed by 160 Filipinos. I lived with five of them—all single men—for five weeks in a shed without windows and infested with giant cockroaches. Under a tin roof and above a garage, we had electricity, water, a toilet, and a locked steel door. It wasn't exactly a slum, but still wretched, loud, and stinking, and we slept on wooden planks.

The Filipino helpers were poverty stricken although educated, which one could recognize by their English language skills. They took me with them on their visits to the prisons, to the youthful gangs and street children, and to the red-light districts, where they ran a tea room at night. What I experienced there shocked me to my depths. Need existed in Basel and London too, but Manila was in a different league. Children and entire families literally lived in the streets, in the dirt. For the first time I encountered people who were forced to suffer real hunger and humiliation, who were ignored by society, or who were maltreated as underpaid workers and were forced to fight for their right to life on a daily basis. I saw child labor, beggars, and prostitution. Earlier, I seemed to have suppressed that there were people who actually physically suffered from hunger. That didn't fit in my theology. This encounter with the poor almost cost me my belief in a merciful God.

Soon I earned the trust of a few Filipinos who worked with the Mission. Besides their fervor on behalf of the very poor, I also sensed reservations and even smoldering bitterness because of the deep economic chasm between the missionaries from the USA and Canada and themselves, the Filipinos. It was grotesque: Some white workers drove to meetings in their brand new all-terrain vehicles, while the Philippine workers did not even receive their legally required minimum wage and benefits payments. A few years later the missionary organization was sued by the Philippine workers, lost the case, and was forced to give up its ministry. Some of their work was carried on by Filipinos and expat missionaries under a different name.

Servants' approach to the mission was entirely different: At the end of my practicum, I visited three families and a couple of single people from New Zealand and Australia who, under contract to Servants, *lived* in the middle of various slums in Manila. I stayed overnight with them twice in their corrugated tin huts and took part in their time together at a guest house outside the slums. I could not disengage from what I heard there. The Servants had fun together on one hand, but on the other, descriptions of upsetting experiences were exchanged. There was true togetherness—with room for brutal honesty and debate, for consolation and prayer. I was persuaded without reservation to join in their effort to share the conditions of the poor in the slums.

The Servants didn't have a grandiose program such as the North American missionary organization. Instead they learned the language of the Filipinos and formed friendships with their neighbors in the slums. There were modest self-help projects and worship meetings in three small new congregations. Everything was unpretentious and experimental, and often they encountered setbacks. But they were in the truest sense of the word "servants." They took time and valued their engagement not just financially. And they dreamed that God would change things. This togetherness seemed to me to be a kind of "Jesus way."

Back in Switzerland, my impressions were reported accordingly, and they accomplished the desired effect. One year later I said goodbye to the Evangelical Community Basel and to my friends in the CVJM at a beautiful worship service. They assured me that I was to be their "extended arm" to the poor. I felt a solemn momentousness.

First I flew to New Zealand for a seven-week course for slum workers. Thereafter, it was on to the Philippines.

And here I am now, on June 9, 1988, in a narrow partition under a tin roof in a vast slum near Manila.

Blessed are those who receive

"*Gusto kong matuto ng Tagalog, dahil gusto kong maging kaibigan ninyo.*" My language helper, Nardo, the oldest son of my host family, the Opiasas, taught me this sentence: "I would like to learn Tagalog so that I can become your friend."

For weeks now, I've been going from shack to shack repeating this short sentence and causing much merriment. I've imitated and repeated the strange words, but apparently I sound very odd; in any case, my listeners find me highly amusing. But I have to struggle on, because the language is the most important thing right now. It is a hard and fast rule in the Servants group that during the first year no aid programs or projects should be initiated in order to concentrate solely on learning Tagalog, the Filipino language, and seeking genuine relationships not built on aid and projects.

I am relieved about the good humor and lightheartedness of the locals. For them, I represent the strong and rich white man who is supposed to "help" the little brown man. But now they're standing in front of one of these "Amerikanos," as they call us, and are surprised to realize that he doesn't bring any help at all. On the contrary, even he is dependent on help—on *their* help! Now *they* are the experts, *they* know the language, *they* know how one navigates through life here. They enjoy the role reversal and gladly help me. In contrast, I don't always find it easy to endure my helplessness. Often I find myself tense because I have too little privacy and too much noise around me. I encounter injustice, sickness, and death everywhere I go. I feel powerless and frustrated, react loudly or impatiently, or withdraw, disheartened. People sense how overwhelmed and vulnerable I am. This builds trust—and friendships.

Yesterday three persistent young *baklas*, homosexual transvestites, deliberately pursued me and came on to me. "You are so handsome... I want to marry you... come on... let's just have some fun...." I had a lot of trouble getting rid of them. And suddenly I felt something of the humiliation that a woman degraded to a sex object is subjected to. In these first few weeks I have already experienced many unexpected situations that sent me reeling.

As I continue my walk, for some reason a tiny shack attracts my attention. I glance inside: It's dark and damp and reeks of excrement and urine. "What a filthy hole," flashes through my mind. Then, in the midst of the muck, I discover three children, the smallest about two, the oldest at most five-years-old. They are malnourished and neglected. No parents in sight. Horrified, I run to Nanay Opiasa and ask her what's going on with the children.

"The father is an alcoholic, he's abandoned the mother."

"And where is the mother?"

"She probably couldn't stand to see her children go hungry and ran away too, with the youngest baby."

I shudder. "But who will feed the children now? Did you see their little bellies bloated from hunger?"

"Well, we neighbors stop in now and then and give them something to eat. We feel sorry for them too, damn it. That father should be killed!"

"Nanay, the children won't last long like this."

Nanay reads my thoughts and finally says, "Alright, bring them here. We don't have any room but until we find a new place for them...."

Regarding "in the first year, only language" policy... the first month seems much too long for me. They can't demand that I look the other way! As a medically trained professional care provider, I'm accustomed to saving lives. Therefore I allow myself again and again to help a little, to provide vital medications, rice, or milk powder. But it's like opening a can of worms. On one hand, I'm a "helper" again, on the other hand, the neighbors want me to help them too. Jealousy is a big problem here and can have dangerous consequences.

So I force myself to bear the pressure as best I can and to hold myself back from offering aid. I simply listen and share the pain in silence. At least I'm allowed to pray for people. Here everyone believes in God, and they consider prayer to be a concrete form of devotion and empathy. That I am able to pray for them probably does me as much good as it does them.

Noriel, the Teenager

Last night I discovered how the Opiasa parents manage to sleep together on the narrow sofa under the little awning in front of the shack without falling off: They lie opposite one another, with their feet next to the other's head. I have never understood why the Opiasas also share their house with a variety of pets. It's already crowded enough.

When they have guests it becomes even more crowded and guests come by quite often. Then Noriel, one of the teenagers to whom the pets belong, stretches out to sleep with me on the plank bed under the tin roof. Or he comes up because one of the two fans in the house is aimed toward my cot and provides some relief from the heat of the summer night. Then he sleeps soundly, while I continually wake up to disentangle myself from one of his arms or legs. As a European, this closeness is something to which I have to become accustomed, whereas for single Filipino men it's such a matter of course that they even have a name for it: *Makitulog* (sleeping together). But despite *makitulog* and the confined space, in these five weeks since my arrival, Noriel has found a place in my heart. He is a cheerful boy, always ready for some prank or joke.

Today my language helper, Nardo, and his wife, Jovelyn, baptized their baby, Jonar. I missed the celebration, however, because I attended a team meeting of Servants in town. Upon my return, Noriel is sitting under a window opening and staring dolefully into space. Normally in this state of mind he has his best friend, his dog, with him. Now, however, he is alone.

"*Bakit,*" I ask, "why"? Noriel swallows. I sit down next to him and put my arm protectively around his shoulders.

"They ate my dog," he says, and breaks into tears.

They actually served up this filthy, sick mongrel dog as a feast in honor of little Jonar's baptism. They first hid the truth from Noriel, but it wasn't long before he figured out where the meat came from. I shuddered. Thank heavens I wasn't here for the celebration. I would have had to partake of the meat, and with every bite I would have seen the ailing old animal in front of me. On the other hand, the people here desperately need protein, and meat is a great luxury.

Noriel sobbed without restraint. I held him tight for a little while. Perhaps this loss had opened an old wound in him. He told me some time ago how they resisted the forced move to Bagong Silang three years ago, in the inner-city slum where he grew up. Together with the neighbors they erected barricades against the armed bands of landowners who preceded the bulldozers to overcome the resistance of the slum dwellers with batons and guns, and chased them away so that the bulldozers could barrel over their shacks. It turned into a bloody battle against the armed throng at the time, with two dead among the wounded. One of the victims was a teenager who bled to death from a gunshot wound—Noriel's best friend.

What happens to a person who even as a teenager has to suffer one loss after another? That night I fall asleep exhausted and deep in thought.

Ana and Rodelio

I stroll past an open shack and smile at a young mother, cooking. "*Kain tayo*," she calls out to me cheerfully, and invites me to stay and eat. "*Salamat*," I answer, declining politely. But there's no reason that I shouldn't try out a few Tagalog sentences on her while she's cooking.

Somehow I manage to get this across to her and she says, in surprisingly good English, "No problem, I am Ana, go ahead." Whoever speaks English here happily makes it known. English implies good breeding and is evidence of a good education. And Ana wants to seize the opportunity—me—to practice her English.

As our mutual language lesson proceeds, Ana again extends her invitation to stay for the meal. Her gesture is unmistakable, and I have no chance to escape, so I accept. Ana serves a thin rice soup, and I suspect that it is the entire meal for this very poor family. The children cavorting about are sweet but incredibly thin. "At least they seem to be healthy," flits through my mind.

While we're slurping hot soup and amusing ourselves watching the children having fun, a young woman suddenly thrusts her head in the door, which is wide open—very important when a single man and a young woman are in the same room.

"Father!" the children shout with one voice. "Look, the Amerikano here is our new friend." Now I realize that the pretty and heavily made-up woman's face with matching hairstyle belongs to a young man, who is apparently the father of the family. Naturally I hide my surprise.

"This is Rodelio," Ana introduces me to her husband, as if his dressing up as a woman were the most normal thing in the world. "He's coming from the city, directly from his work."

That evening, I tell my host family about my strange encounter.

"The father was unable to find work except as a woman, so he transformed himself into a woman for work," old Mother Opiasa explains. "What kind of work?" I ask and realize at the same moment how naïve I am. Nanay sighs deeply and slowly says, "When children go hungry, many parents are willing to do any kind of work."

I'm still pondering this remark, lying on my wooden bed that evening. The children are hungry, but if an Amerikano passes by, even the poorest Filipinos invite him in with a *kain tayo*, "let us eat together." When someone repeats *kain tayo* at least three times, then the invitation is sincerely meant and it would be very impolite to refuse.

Even the most primitive shacks in the slum are often kept painstakingly clean inside. And while the surroundings are usually anything but clean, as a guest I am obliged to remove my shoes before I enter. Normally water to drink is offered. If I refuse because of concern regarding contamination, the host will quickly round up a cola from the nearest *sari-sari*, as the small family-run stores located on every corner are called. For this he'll readily run up a debt without further thought, if necessary. To host a stranger is very important to him.

If I can anticipate and foresee this implicit obligation of my host, I do well to quickly obtain a large cola and a few fruits myself, preferably for the whole family. That is called *pasalubong*, and means "hostess gift." Do some people hope that such a gift will be forthcoming when they issue the invitation? Could be. But in view of their miserable living conditions, I wouldn't hold it against them. In any case, I find their spontaneous hospitality genuine and impressive.

Jonar's Death

I have now been in Bagong Silang for seven weeks. It is time for a short return to the Servants house. We slum workers from the West must reappear now and again to get some air; to bear the misery without interruption would be too much to ask. This time I'll be away for three days.

Before I leave, I explain to Nardo and Jovelyn how they should prepare and dispense the antidehydration solution, Orisol, as a precaution, since Jonar has a light case of diarrhea. Diarrhea is not unusual among infants. Jonar is being suckled, he is well nourished with full cheeks, often laughing and bubbly, full of life, the sunshine within the shack. But safe is safe. And now, I'm out of here!

The Servants house is an oasis for all of us. We unload and fill our emotional tanks. The house serves as our official address, replete with telephone, fax, and a safe for passports and papers. A secretary and a housekeeper free us from mundane responsibilities; together with a couple who are in charge of house administration, they provide us slum workers with a little bit of home, making themselves available for conversation and visits and provide the possibility of overnight accommodations.

We are approximately twenty slum workers altogether, families with children as well as single people from New Zealand, Australia, and England. Every few weeks we meet here, listen to one another, laugh and cry, and encourage one another. The degree of misery that confronts us pushes us to our limits, and brings the best and worst to the surface in everyone. One gains insight into the interior world of others and allows others entry into one's own interior world. This forthrightness and trust are liberating and supportive, no one needs to pretend, and feigned strengths and principles soon crumble in the face of reality. Sometimes it happens that tired or burned-out colleagues are compelled to take a long vacation—or to finally return home. New workers are provided particularly intensive care.

We follow various rituals in our house—praying is one of them, and often also a short lecture on the Bible. Denominational differences do not matter at all; in light of the reality of this place, it would be meaningless. We celebrate that which we have in common and thereby admit our differences.

As it is, we are all dependent, also financially. We live on the support of the friends and church congregations in our homelands. The idea is that we share everything with one another, just as the first Christians. In the meantime, I'm no longer surprised that this actually works, whether regarding private expenses or project costs. We discuss what it actually means to live "in moderation" again and again.

The Lord's Supper is prepared by an Australian this time, with chips and cola. A break in tradition—rather unusual for me, but I'm more than sure that Jesus Christ is also present; he smiles and is pleased. Missing is a Catholic brother: He absents himself from communion from time to time to remind us how painful the rupture between the various branches of Christianity really is. Other issues are of far greater concern to me. But I am glad that he allows me to share his perception, as I share mine with him. Thus we progress together.

We laugh a lot in these three days, eat well, and even make a short excursion. Adequately rested, I plunge back into "my shack" in "my" slum. But just as I want to greet my host family happily, I gasp for air. At the wall where Nardo and Jovelyn normally sleep, Jonar is lying—on a funeral bier.

Numb, I sit down on the lone wooden bench and stare at the white, bloated little face of the tiny corpse. "We did everything according to the directions," Nardo and Jovelyn assure me without my asking. "But the dysentery became worse and Jonar noticeably weaker. Then we raced with him the great distance to the hospital in the city, but it was too late."

This can't have happened. Not in "my" family! I feel as if I've been lamed; I can't even weep. This doesn't escape Nardo's notice, and then he actually says: "Jesus loves Jonar so much that he took him for himself." Now he comforts me, of all things—he comforts me, rather than my comforting him.

After the first shock, I'm overcome with rage about an incapable and cynical government that moves—no, maroons—people in a place where there is no clean water and no work, no means to live. And about the whole world, that allows this misery to continue without doing anything, and about the hundred-thousand Christians of this city, whose Christianity consists of sitting it out in their air conditioned middle-class churches!

The dead child lies in the house for nine days. Relatives from the provinces arrive. All are supposed to be able to mourn copiously and to say goodbye. The little coffin is closed; one can only still see the dead child through a small glass window. They injected formaldehyde into the little body to delay its decomposition. Nonetheless, I detect the odor of decay.

A few wilted flowers lie on the table next to a burning candle and an open box for donations. The money is intended to help the family with burial costs. In front of the shack, the Opiasas have stretched a fabric awning with ropes, so that the visitors and the neighbors are protected from the sun during the day and from the dew at night. The neighbors are running an almost uninterrupted game of chance under the awning. A portion of the proceeds goes to the family in mourning. The atmosphere is strange. People weep and laugh, play and drink the entire night until dawn. Only Jovelyn sits and stares ahead, as if she weren't present. Now and then, she emits a loud sob.

During the days of mourning, the floor may not be swept. If this dictum is ignored, another member of the family will follow the deceased and will also die. The family members are actually not supposed to sleep, according to an old animistic tradition, although few adhere to this. The bereaved family members are also not supposed to wash themselves. The Opiasa siblings, Mina, Dario,

Berna, and Noriel don't hold to this either, which doesn't disturb me in the least. . . . Apparently the three active Christians from my friend Rob's Living Spring Fellowship have set aside their fear of spirits and are here, in order to free themselves from their subjection to animism. With their guitar in accompaniment, they sing solemn and joyful songs again and again and bring some light into the oppressive atmosphere.

I feel tired and sick, and have caught a cold . . . an absurd word in this heat. But I've received a gift from heaven at the right time, in the person of my Swiss friend Christian Auer, who has arrived for a whole week's visit. He is a student at the Swiss Tropical Institute and in conjunction with his thesis research will dedicate himself to the "Smoky Mountains," a particularly horrible slum, where he will investigate parasites and the vaccine situation in children. Conversation with Christian and a prayer together does me good. They help me to properly mourn. And so I manage more or less to get over the worst of it.

My Little Clinic

Middle of August. Nine Weeks. And forty three more to go before my language-learning year, in keeping with the iron-clad rules of Servants is over, and I can dedicate myself to my "actual" work. But except for the iron-clad rules, what would stand in the way of already beginning my "actual" work in a small way? To work as a community nurse in the slums would actually enhance my language lessons!

"Hey, Rob, listen, what would you think of a little walk-in clinic? A health-maintenance service that I could offer at least two days each week?"

Rob and Lorraine are not at all enthusiastic about my suggestion. But they know only too well how difficult it is to concentrate on trying to learn the language rather than dealing with the urgent needs that confront us daily. And they know how good it feels to be able to do something. When I consider Lorraine's kindergarten, in which many children are being prepared for grade school, and her nutrition program in which 108 of 220 undernourished children have already reached their normal weight in the first year. . . .

Before my arrival, Joan, an older Servants colleague, had maintained a kind of bandage and salve clinic. After her return to New Zealand, there was a void, which Rob and Lorraine had noticed. "I could better concentrate on language learning on the other days," I assured Rob, "and on those days I wouldn't always help the sick neighbors immediately; rather, I would refer them to the clinic instead."

After some back-and-forth discussion, Rob and Lorraine agreed. I am ecstatic! The work awaits—there's no hospital and hardly any doctors in the area. A private physician worked here—for pay—until just a few weeks ago, until he lost his life due to an "electrocution," as the slum dwellers describe it when someone taps an electrical line illegally and makes a mistake....

Just days later, we're ready: "My" clinic is furnished, a humble shack with a corrugated tin roof. I stand in the center and sweat. On the left is a translator, on the right an open handbook with the apt title, *Where There is No Doctor.* Rudimentary surgical instruments for the care of wounds, a gas cooker for their sterilization, blood pressure apparatus, an otoscope, a box of medications for pain and fever, various antibiotics, antidiarrhea medicines, disinfection solutions, bandages, and quite a lot of salves and creams. It is an unintended comical sight. There is, of course, little to laugh at, given the reality of the needs of the people waiting outside. The queue is long, and I am overwhelmed by the great demand.

One learns. In the first few days of operation I see that some patients bring medical prescriptions with them. They had apparently found a government doctor somewhere, working gratis, who examined them and gave them the prescription without bothering to determine whether they could afford to pay for the medications (which was probably never a possibility). Most of the time, these doctors prescribed more or less the same three things: A pain and fever reducer, an expensive vitamin, and an even more expensive antibiotic. It's a bad joke: Instead of the expensive prescription, the people could obtain the prescribed vitamin by eating relatively inexpensive little citrus fruits, the *kalamansi,* or indigenous vegetables.

On the other hand, antibiotics are relatively easy to come by, in any measure and without prescription, but also without any directions regarding the appropriate application. Many patients therefore don't follow a course of antibiotic treatment, but rather simply swallow two or three tablets. Instead of getting well quickly, they slowly become resistant to the antibiotics, which sooner or later stop working. A lot of instruction is clearly needed.

We're a good team: Berna, Isabel, and Cris—three young people from the Living Spring Fellowship—as well as Lorraine and I. Over time, something resembling a system develops in our clinic: Outside while the queue waits, there are prayers and instruction regarding medications; inside there is treatment. The very ill are treated first, and in the afternoon we provide a vehicle that transports emergency patients to the city hospital. The little project is financed by European donors whom I keep informed by sending regular update letters. I often remember what my friends in the Evangelical Community Basel (EGB) and the CVJM told me upon my departure: That I was their extended arm to the poor.

A young boy is carried into the clinic. He has large open wounds on both feet, third-degree burns, and of course they are filthy and infected. "How in heaven's name did this happen?" I ask, frightened. "The child was hungry, often screamed, and often brawled with his siblings," my interpreter says. "His father was drunk, lost his temper, poured gasoline on his feet, and struck a match."

I gasp for air. "We have to take the children away from him," I say, enraged, "one can't absolve him of blame here!"

"Don't worry," my interpreter explains. "The man has been taken to task. When the neighbors learned of the incident, they beat him half to death. He'll take better care of his children now."

In the evening I visit the family. I step into a wooden shed onto a damp, bare mud floor and find an open lath-board for sleeping, two fiber mats, a plastic bucket for water, and a charcoal cooker. And I see two little children and a completely emaciated mother with an infant suckling at her breast. As I leave the hut, I break into tears.

Even though I'm only in the clinic three days per week, I soon notice how the work is beginning to devour me. Opening abscesses, pulling infected teeth, treating and stitching up wounds, bathing rashes, doing battle with worms, lowering fevers, sometimes with success, sometimes without, and sometimes not knowing what will happen to the patient at all. Often I have the feeling that we really have to fight to achieve our successes. All the better when we have the opportunity to share in them—as with Jolli.

The ten-year-old came to us with burns on her stomach and abdomen. Our treatment with silver sulfate seemed to have a good effect. Nevertheless, she suffered a setback: Suddenly Jolli didn't want to eat anymore although she was undernourished even before. We took her to the hospital where she quickly recovered. Since then we have regularly provided her with medications to fight tuberculosis. The treatment is working; Jolli is finally gaining weight. And she is smiling again.

That the clinic would be helpful in my efforts to learn the language is, naturally, an illusion. Nonetheless, I have contact with many families and their tragedies at these appointments. I learn a lot and again and again am confronted with limits. Often patients appear for whom no medical help is available under our particular circumstances. Sometimes, in my helplessness, I take photos of strange illnesses and forward them with additional explanations to my personal physician in Switzerland.

Most of the people who receive treatment from us never return. Sometimes that depresses me. Today, before the Sunday service, however, a mother approaches and thanks me for saving her child's life. I am overjoyed. Such rare follow-up compensates for the long and difficult days.

Later, in the chapel, another mother proudly introduces her six-year-old daughter to the people gathered together, and reports that God had miraculously healed her. I remember the child; five days earlier she was brought to us with bloody, festering abscesses on her head and stomach. We laid on hands and prayed for healing. And now the little one stands before us, her fresh scars bearing witness to her unusually fast recovery. If we could only experience such gifts from God more often!

Mrs. Mercy

I have lost my language helper: Nardo and his wife, Jovelyn, have gone away. Quietly, they've left our resettlement area and have returned to the province where the family lived as fishermen for generations. Mother Opiasa is sad, naturally, but I can understand why Nardo and Jovelyn took this step. They lost Jonar, their only child, just a few weeks ago, and the haunting scene in the shack with the tiny corpse on its bier has not only been burned into *my* mind. I wouldn't be able to bear this shack and this death-inducing poverty any longer either. Now Nardo and Jovelyn want to begin a new life elsewhere. I hope they'll be able to do so.

Each person who leaves the resettlement area is replaced by ten new ones. Almost every day, within sight of my new home, rusty yellow trucks drive by, with "Demolition Team" painted on the side. The pickup trucks stop and spew out the families they've transported. Today I heard it's supposed to be about two-hundred people. Rob heads in that direction, and I go with him.

The group of transplants are a sorry sight. They sit there, with large eyes, thirsty, and with empty stomachs, on the meager belongings that they could salvage and the remains of their former slum dwellings in the inner city—wooden planks and corrugated metal.

A well-nourished lady steps onto a wooden crate and introduces herself as Mrs. "Mercy" . . . right! Rob is familiar with this scenario: Mrs. Mercy is the representative of the local government and will officially welcome the new arrivals, while the slum in which these people lived until just a few hours ago is being demolished by bulldozers.

"I admit that as yet we have no water," Mrs. Mercy laughs, a little embarrassed, "and electricity is also still absent, at least at the moment. But instead we have a lot of fresh air here, in contrast to Manila." A few people laugh, although I don't quite comprehend why. Do they sense the embarrassment of the "important lady," and laugh good naturedly at her grim humor? Do they envy or admire her? Don't they notice the cynicism?

"Now I am able to introduce to you our new livelihood project," trumpets the woman with the colorful chubby cheeks, to the crowd: "All who are willing will be trained in the crafting of Christmas angels, for export to Germany!" She lifts a Christmas angel into the air: "In five weeks you can earn up to two *pesos* per hour!"

Nobody is laughing any more. I gasp for air. Eight hours of crafting Christmas angels yields 4.5 pounds of subsidized rice. I have an urge to forcibly remove Mrs. Mercy from her perch on the wooden crate. What these deportees really want to know is how one can build a shelter without decent construction materials and with an empty stomach. It's June, and the rainy season lasts until October.

"Rob!" I say, "if we could at least give this group a little welcome gift? Some rice and milk powder? I could take the money from the donor account of Servants Switzerland! We could at least help them survive through the first few weeks."

Rob ponders my suggestion. "It may only be assistance at the outset and not more," he finally explains. "We may not in any way foster long-term dependence."

Later I regret my suggestion. For strategic reasons, Rob doesn't want to go around Mrs. Mercy, who represents the government, and entrusts the money for the purchase of the emergency rations to her. Mrs. Mercy disappears with the money and is never seen again. I am reminded that in this slum there are many opportunities to learn from one's mistake. Finally we are able to help the new arrivals nonetheless—this time with trustworthy friends, who live here themselves. Rob has some experience with self-help projects, and I will gain some—that's clear.

"Give the hungry man a fish and he will be sated for a day; teach him to fish and he'll never be hungry again." I admit that this sounds very wise. And that the statement is quite insightful has in the meantime been discussed, especially in Europe. But later one stands in Bagong Silang and asks oneself, how one is supposed to teach someone who is starving, or alcohol dependent, or very sick, to fish ... and someone who has no fishing tackle, not to mention that he doesn't have a license to fish in the lake, which doesn't belong to him. The fishing license belongs to a corrupt official in this land, and the lake belongs to a satiated owner who is surrounded by a hungry crowd that wants permission to fish. And if one of the hungry ones becomes one of the satiated because he's acquired a lake, then he'll most likely behave similarly. Like Val, the basket-maker, whom Rob described to me on the way home.

Val visited Rob's Christian congregation, where Rob gave him the name of a rattan exporter whom he could contact in Manila. Rob even provided him a loan for start-up capital. Val hired two basket-makers and began production. Soon he had ten workers, a full belly, and paid his credit-payments punctually. But Val began to treat his workers worse and worse. Their starvation wages were far below the minimum existential wage. There were always enough desperate people in Bagong Silang who were prepared to do such slave work. Once Val had paid off the start-up capital, he never returned to the congregation. "I had hoped that Val would acquire a sense of duty," Rob says. "Building a value system is a central task in every good course of development. And I don't want any people at our Christian Fellowship who hope only to receive material help, or like Val, only come to the service because they feel obligated to me as their lender."

Apparently uncompromising capitalism functions not only in the global economy but also in the slum. Rather than sharing material things with one another, I think we should share life. No one guarantees, however, that this kind of life is important to another and animates him with goodness. Besides, it's not so easy to separate the one from the other; the life one should share with another also includes loaves and fishes.

Mrs. "Mercy" from the government and Val, the capitalist, will occupy my thoughts for some time to come.

Jolli

It's only ten o'clock in the morning but already burning hot. There's not the slightest breath of wind. Of course the fans aren't moving again and haven't been for two weeks. Too many settlers have illegally tapped into the electrical lines and overloaded the transformers, which burned out. And since no one here can pay the bills, no new transformers will be installed.

I sit on my wooden cot and repeat, repeat, repeat the Tagalog sentence with the new vocabulary words. It's enough to drive one to tears or to swear. I'll never get these words into my dim brain, and without new words I can forget about progress, because without practice I'll never learn this language, and if I don't learn it, then I can't accomplish anything here, and if I can't achieve anything, what am I doing here? I, of all people?

When I was fifteen, my French teacher chased me out of class and down the corridors of the school, shouting that I was a language idiot and would never learn a foreign language, and that he didn't want to see me in his class again; and on my final report card, a grade for French was indeed missing. Nonetheless, in the three years in England, I passed all the language exams in English. But English isn't Tagalog, and in England I had a bed instead of a wooden plank, and fresh air!

Everywhere mosquito bites, old ones and fresh ones. And then these stupid ants. In all colors and sizes. Sometimes you can feel them crawling across your back. Most of the time it's only drops of sweat, gliding slowly down to the base of your spine. It's hot, and it itches. It always itches where one can't reach with one's hand. A million neon signs glow in the shopping districts of this megacity, and out here, we don't even have the electricity for fans. It's enough to make one cry.

Jolli has also died—she, of all people, who for some time now, could smile again. Last Sunday, she was at the fellowship meeting. She had a fever, and I advised her parents to take her to the hospital. She died there two days later. She caught the grippe, the doctors said.

The fellow from the funeral home really infuriated me. He demanded 2,600 *pesos* for transporting the corpse, embalming and burial, although it was clear to him that Jolli's father would never, for the life of him, be able to get this money together. He is unemployed and hardly knows how to provide food for his three remaining children and his wife. Twenty-six thousand *pesos* are two months' wages for a service worker. By begging, they were able to gather only 300 pesos and couldn't properly bury Jolli, her mother sobbed.

We could help Jolli's family, but what about all the others? One is so powerless out here. It is a dead end for body and soul. One becomes enraged. *I* become enraged! And yet I have it much better than the Filipinos. In contrast to them, I'm living here voluntarily. And when I really can't stand it any longer, I get into an open Jeepney, hold a cloth over my nose, and after forty minutes of bouncing and dust, I'm in the next municipal quarter, in an air conditioned restaurant or cinema. I have the spare change for this. It is only somewhat helpful in learning the language, but it gives me some air, some distance from Bagong Silang, where already at ten o'clock in the morning it is scorching hot and all the fans stand idle once again. I don't know how the people here can stand it.

Actually, I do know how: They are stronger than I am.

Death in the Chapel

Sunday. Morning service at Rob's Living Spring Christian Fellowship. The diminutive church looks quite solid—too solid for my taste, in comparison to the shacks of some of the members, which consist in part of plastic awnings and cartons. "We simply had to erect a chapel, the people wanted it," Rob explains; "the House of God is much more important to many people here than their own roofs over their heads." He should know. The building provides some additional worthwhile services, functioning as a school and a maternity center.

About thirty adults are at the Sunday service, many mothers with their babies, and approximately twice as many children and a couple of dogs. Next to me stands Nick, one of the few better educated residents of Bagong Silang. He studied architecture, but now works as a technical draftsman and is happy just to have a job. Since they chose the thirty-year-old bachelor as vice president of a small self-help neighborhood organization, he attends the services of the Living Spring Christian Fellowship. He has a pleasant, quiet demeanor that one doesn't find here all too often.

People come and go, but that doesn't seem to disturb anyone. It is oppressively hot under the tin roof on the crude cement bricks. We're sitting shoulder to shoulder on wooden planks. It smells. Hygiene is a luxury here, soap and water in short supply. Drinking water has to be bought in bottles or canisters, and people stand in long lines for water to bathe and wash.

The door and the window of the chapel are wide open. May one hope to catch a small breath of fresh air? Or does one wish to include the neighborhood in the activities of the gathering? The only fan is trained on Rob, who stands tall in front, in the Filipino dress of a Philippine man, the *barong*, and with pearls of sweat on his forehead, leads the congregants.

We sing hymns about God and his love. The devotion of the people touches me—some have come without breakfast in their stomachs. After the hymns and a reading from the Bible, Rob gives a simple sermon and invites visitors to come forward along with a group of indigenous faithful so that they could also be included in prayer. Much movement and noise ensues, since almost everyone pushes to get to the front. Where need is so obvious, no one has to conceal it. Individuals sob. I believe, nonetheless, that I sense joy, enmeshed in the tears of misery.

Rob embraces a woman. In her arms she holds a child enveloped in a white cloth, her four-year-old son who is skin and bones. I know the family through my little clinic; a poor fishing family, who arrived in the capital city a few weeks ago with the hope of finding work and assistance, but who finally were stranded here in the slum like so many others. The father has trouble walking; the four children are terribly malnourished.

"Let us pray!" Rob calls out. "The child is very, very sick, only a miracle can help here." We pray, in an undertone. After a while, it becomes quiet. Suddenly, the mother cries out. The cry cuts me to the quick. Rob bends over the child. Then he says, "The boy is dead."

A lump rises in my throat. Just last week two small children died in the adjacent neighborhood. One of the impoverished fathers put together a wood casket, dug a hole in the earth next to the cemetery, and "buried" the child there. He didn't have the money for a plot within the cemetery, where the deceased are immured according to Philippine custom. Most of the bereaved survivors can't pay for a priest either.

Sometimes, when I'm alone at night, I scream at God. Often I get no answer, as in the past week.

The following week I am again sitting in Rob's little church, when to my great surprise the mother of the child who had died the previous week arrives at the chapel. She says that her son had already for some time not wanted to eat anything, nor could he, and he also couldn't speak any more. On that morning, however, he awakened and said clearly and distinctly, "Mother, take me to church, I want to go to church with you today."

For the mother and the believers it was clear: The dying child knew that he was going to God's eternity, accompanied by a congregation praying for him. For me, this message from the mother about the wish of the dying child was an alleviation of my misgivings. Perhaps God's eternal world is better for the child than Bagong Silang, which is so hostile to life. In such an ending to a tragic event, I can find some consolation. . . .

Nardo, the Resistance Fighter

Mama Opiasa is worried. Not only have Nardo and Jovelyn left Bagong Silang, but now we've also heard that Nardo has left Jovelyn and moved to the mountains. With her hand covering her mouth, Mama Opiasa confides in me that he has most likely joined the NPA. The New People's Army is the armed branch of the illegal Marxist Party in the Philippines whose leadership has been living in exile in Holland for many years. But the approximately 24,000 fighters are waging a bloody and unsuccessful guerilla war that resulted in ten thousand dead in the last years. The government troops pursue the NPA fighters with great hostility, and to be related to an NPA fighter is extremely risky.

Since Nardo isn't here any longer, the second-oldest, Dario, has assumed the role of the *panganay*, the first-born son, who comes right after the father in the hierarchy of the family. Dario is twenty-years-old. We both have spoken often about visiting the hometown of the Opiasas, the little town of Daet, located in Camarines Norte, a province of the Philippine administrative area called Bicolandia, directly on the ocean. "It's extraordinarily beautiful there," Dario enthuses, beaming.

There are three reasons to undertake this trip now: Mama Opiasa's concern about Nardo, Dario's homesickness for the carefree years of his childhood, and my urgent need for time out. We'll combine, therefore, a vacation week at the seashore with the search for the missing man. This kind of pragmatism, which in wealthy Western Europe would seem cynical, doesn't bother me at all anymore. The trip by bus would take ten fatiguing hours. Instead, we take an airplane, since inland flights are cheap, and the time we save will actually accrue toward the vacation.

In just over an hour's flight we arrive in Daet. It is beautiful, idyllic, pristine—a completely different world. I am as enraptured as Dario, who is effervescent with joy, and, as a proud tour guide, shows me everything that the dreamy fishing village offers: Running every morning on glorious sandy beaches a mile long; swimming in the clear, lukewarm ocean; fishing in a paddle boat; allowing one's soul to flourish; living in a simple little bamboo hut under coconut palms—what could be more beautiful?

"Dario," I ask him, "explain to me why in the world your parents left this place?"

Since Dario knows Bagong Silang, he sees the beauty of Daet as clearly as I do. But because he lived here a few years, he also recognizes the dark and light aspects of the province. "You know," he says, "nothing moves here except the sea and the palms in the wind. With a little exertion and a little luck you can fill your belly with fruits and fish, but otherwise you don't make any headway. You can't earn any money here, and there's not enough land for all the children and their families. Since the industrial fisheries deplete the coves, there's not enough as there was earlier. Sometimes the guerillas of the NPA come into the villages and levy "war taxes," a kind of protection money. And when they don't come, then the government soldiers arrive and torment the people because they suspect them of harboring guerillas."

"But, despite everything, isn't that still better than Bagong Silang?"

"The young people who move away from here don't dream of Bagong Silang!" No, of course not; Dario is right. "They dream of Manila, of sports competitions, concerts, movies, and limitless opportunities. What do you think, why do all the rich people live in the capital? Manila is the door to the great world beyond! In Manila you can find employment brokers, who'll send you abroad to other lands where you can earn dollars to buy a house and a car or at least a refrigerator or television. And if one of the children does well in school, then he or she needs the schools in Manila to get ahead in life. Here in Daet, nobody finds great success."

Neither Dario nor I need to say that most people don't find great success in Manila either, and eventually end up in the slums. We both know that and are therefore enjoying this week at the ocean all the more. More than once, I think about the potential of this region. I see miles of undeveloped land. If these people could get ahead by growing vegetables, by farming, or by breeding animals, they wouldn't have to seek their fortune in Manila, only to die there because of contaminated water. What's needed are developers, investors, capital, and patience.

At the end of our vacation week we set out to search for Nardo, as planned. Dario's aunt provides directions into the mountains of Bicol and gives us cooked rice wrapped in small plastic bags as provisions. We board a bus in Daet; the trip is horrible. The macho Filipino drivers often frighten me more with their break-neck speeding than the criminals in the slum. They make me really angry. One reads again and again about dreadful accidents involving these busses, and not without reason. Consequently, I'm overjoyed when Dario and I can finally get off this speeding pile of rust after a very long hour.

We proceed on foot. Just before we leave the asphalt road that serves as a national highway, a convoy of new military trucks with hundreds of heavily armed government soldiers comes toward us from the opposite direction. It appears that the government does not economize on its military budget. After a short march through a banana plantation, we arrive at a wide river. In the water, two stark naked children play under the watchful eyes of their mothers, who are washing clothes at the riverbank, laughing loudly and enjoying themselves. What a contrast to the military convoy. This idyllic picture has a happy effect on me and warms my heart.

A bamboo raft is lying on the riverbank. Dario negotiates a price with the oarsman and we are able to cross to the other side. Once there, we continue on at a rhythmic pace on a well-defined footpath, but not for long: The footpath turns into a narrow silt path, at some places consisting only of the deep furrows made by the runners of the sleds that are dragged through the sludge by water buffalo. Dario takes off his shoes and goes barefoot, and I continually scrape the heavy red clay from the soles of my gym shoes. It's uphill and downhill, through forests of coconut palms and clearings and thickets, and again and again, paths branch off in every conceivable direction. I can only hope that Dario knows where we are and where we want to go.

Time after time, we pass by *barangays,* little villages composed of wretched straw huts, some with plywood walls, some with walls constructed of crude cement bricks called "hollow blocks." Here there is no electricity; instead, they've fashioned sooty gasoline lamps from beer bottles. Again and again, we meet curious, laughing children, some of whom look quite dirty and neglected and have resorted to begging. Once, twice, three times, Dario briefly speaks with the Filipinos in the local dialect, Bicolano, which I don't understand. I think he's asking them for directions. And then we set off again.

Suddenly, after a seemingly interminable march of about three-hours' duration, a group of armed men appear. As they become aware of us, they advance in our direction, as toward a target. The men are wearing tattered camouflage jackets and look wild and unkempt. I find myself getting scared and can feel my pulse in my throat.

"Keep your camera in your pocket, they're NPA's," Dario hisses at me.

The men surround us. They are carrying automatic weapons and have their fingers on the triggers. "Who are you and what are you looking for here?" one threatens.

"We're looking for my brother, who's disappeared," Dario says.

"And that one?" barks one of the armed men.

"I live with the poor in the slums of Manila," I stammer in a mixture of Tagalog and English, "and fight for justice there, like you—although without weapons; only with the Bible."

One of the men steps toward me. He appears to be the leader. He extends his hand, which is missing two fingers. "It's a pleasure, friend, my name is Sergeant Fox," he says in good English. "We're searching for two missing comrades. Forget that you ran into us." And as quickly as they appeared, they disappear.

We set out again, too. I try to sort out my feelings. The friendly gesture of the leader touched me. Who here is actually the hero and who is the villain? On one side are the Communist guerilla fighters of the hapless New People's Army, on the other side the government troops, who with Western technological weapons protect a corrupt system, which allows a large segment of its people to live below the poverty level, and which nonetheless takes part in profitable economic pacts with the richest nations of the world.

Of course, the demarcation can't be drawn that simply. The good and the bad lie side by side in the heart of each individual, no matter where he stands.

We march another grueling hour in the oppressive heat, until we reach yet another small settlement. And there, in a simple little straw house, we find Nardo. He's overjoyed by our surprise visit, and yet he appears a bit sad. He seems worn-out, his deep-set eyes under his dark locks make him appear years older than he is.

The hut is so small that we all go outside to sit on the mountain grass. It is very quiet. We pry open a couple of tins of sardines and mix the contents with cold cooked rice and drink hot, sweet coffee that Nardo brews for us on a little wood fire. A refreshing breeze blows down from the mountain. Dario tells Nardo all the news about the family, although Nardo is sparing with his words. I have the feeling that he's ashamed that we have found him here alone, without Jovelyn.

"I can't bear life in the city any longer," he says, "I belong here in the hills and the forest." As we tell him about our encounter with the NPA's, he smiles: "You mustn't be afraid of them. I am one of them myself."

Mata, the "Bodyguard"

September 1988. I moved ten days ago, into my own little house with plywood walls and a straw roof. I can connect a lamp and a ventilator to a truck battery. I shed no tears over leaving the hot tin roof at the Opiasas' behind. Besides, it was too intimate at the Opiasas, both externally and internally—like a sitting hen, Mama Opiasa had gained complete control over my life.

A couple of unemployed neighbors who were happy to be able to earn a little money built the shack for me. My own home stands on a parcel of land belonging to James, the son of Mang Kaimo, who lives next door with his wife. Mang Kaimo is one of the oldest members of the Living Spring Fellowship, a fine fellow and a patient advisor to his family and neighbors. In broken English, Mang Kaimo once told me that he was formerly a driver, worked like a dog, chased other women, and when he was drunk, tied up and beat his children so that they would behave. Then six years ago, he found God, who brought love into his life. Since then he hasn't drunk a drop of alcohol. He confessed this to me in the presence of his children.

His story is typical. The conscientious fathers who are responsible and moral, almost without exception, report an encounter with God that restored meaning and dignity to their lives. The others flee from their degrading poverty by turning to alcohol. They dilute the high alcohol content of fusel oil with ice water so that it's easier to swallow. Many are unemployed or addicted to gambling or both: A vicious circle. The mothers thus carry the major burden of the family and function as mothers to their husbands since they have no other choice. As a result, the sons have no exemplary model to emulate.

Now and then, through my earphones, I flee to Antonio Vivaldi, although it is less a flight than taking pleasure in what is beautiful and good in this world. I have the feeling that I'm experiencing what the other Servants term a culture shock. Everything is getting to me. I get upset about everything and nothing, and mostly about myself. My loathsome thoughts about—and reactions to—Filipinos frighten me. Sometimes I catch myself noticing only the resignation, laziness, and superficiality of the people here. Then I feel as if I'm losing a godly perspective, the positive dream, along with the joy of labor and of life.

In the days after my move I watch teenagers who hang around the area, bored and without purpose. I approach them and ask a couple of hesitant questions. They like that, and have all the time in the world for my practical language lessons. To help the Amerikano is cool, and to learn English words from him is even cooler, since English reeks of education, and being educated smells cool. In short, they like me, and I like them. They are incredibly open.

"You have no family, so you need bodyguards," they tell me. "From now on, we are your bodyguards!"

So now I have a villa and also bodyguards. They name my plywood house the "Orphanage." As a matter of fact, three young boys have slept in my hut in the last few nights. Without invitation, between five and ten others have also found a place to sleep by squeezing into the space under my entry awning. Most of them are orphans, or half-orphans; others have run away or been chased away. They're not welcome anywhere, except here.

Sometimes in the evenings we sit under the awning, basking in the glorious colors of twilight before the tropical night falls, accompanied by chirping crickets and barking dogs, almost as in a movie. Some of the boys are very musical. One strums a guitar, others sing or perform well-known songs from all over the world, and their eyes sparkle. Except for Mata—for him, only one eye sparkles. The other was torn from its socket when he was a little boy, playing with firework casings. The other boys call the fifteen-year-old "Mata," meaning "one-eye," although his name is actually Brian.

Mata lives with his two siblings and his mother in a crude cement brick shack with a tamped down mud floor. The open, sometimes purulent wound in his face was apparently the reason why no one found it necessary to send him to school. Instead he was already forced to work as a child, so that his fatherless family had something to eat. Until a week ago, he labored as a day-worker at a construction site, but he developed a fever and his employer chased him away. Mata is here often. We all appreciate him for his genial personality.

Mata is not the only one without a proper education. Several of the other young boys can't read. They have no prospects in life, and they know it. They hunger for a purpose. Again and again, I tell them that there is a God who created them and loves them. Sometimes we read the Bible, they in Tagalog, I in English. Noriel Opiasa is often with us. He knows a little English and often helps me with explanations—my Tagalog is still fragmentary. But I don't need Tagalog to see how deeply touched the young boys are; a look into their eyes suffices.

Despite everything, the situation is not satisfactory. It's not enough to raise their hopes; the boys need prospects. And I need time.

Ruth, the Doctor

I am happy about an interesting interruption to my language studies: My family physician, Dr. Ruth Riner from Riehen, is coming to visit. If everything goes as planned, we will be implementing a medical initiative and vaccination program together with the help of Christians in the region, and at the same time, preaching about Christ. The schedule also includes a few days of team retreats; for

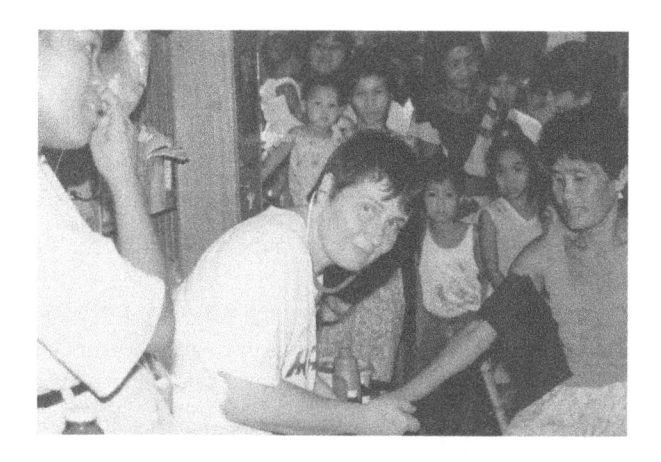

Ruth Riner from Switzerland arrives to offer me some support.

us "slum missionaries," being with a community with whom we have a mutual bond is a necessity of life.

A few days later, it is reality: Ruth arrives, a wonderful, committed woman and a competent doctor. A street that leads to our little clinic runs through Tala, a leper colony. My friends avoid this street, but Ruth does just the opposite. When she hears about the lepers, she asks to visit them.

A hospital and several one-story buildings and barracks serve as shelters for these patients. A village consisting of a large church and a single street with several thousand residents has grown up around the structures. This settlement is overwhelmingly populated by relatives of the lepers, who moved here with the patients in order to be by their side and provide them with most of their essential needs.

Ruth wants to see how the lepers live. As we visit one of the barracks together, we are greeted by a group of approximately forty men. The leprosy bacteria have maimed many of them. Faces, even of the young men, are grotesquely distorted, and some are missing entire limbs.

As we sit with the patients, Ruth raises her skirt. Since an accident she had as a child, she wears a leg prosthesis which she manages so well that one hardly notices that she has only *one* leg of her own. She knocks on the prosthesis and laughs. "I am one of you; I live with a wooden leg, too!"

Ruth, the Caucasian, with her prosthesis and her infectious laugh, instantaneously wins the undivided attention of the men. How quickly understanding and relationships can be created! It's nothing different—other than the intuitive adaptation of the Servants' central principle.

Before Ruth returns to her stressful Swiss family practice, we tack on a couple of days of vacation at the beach. It also does me some good to leave misery behind for a while. I enjoy the vacation islands with Western comfort. And Boracay delivers what the advertisements promise: From the fine-grained white sand one can pleasantly allow oneself to slowly slip into the crystal clear tropical seawater; evenings, one can slurp fruit shakes and listen to the melancholy sounds of the talented soloists on the beach.

After these relaxing days we have to make an immense effort to head to the airport. There is a three-hour ride over unpaved, bumpy roads in an overcrowded Jeepney. I manage to get an airy place to sit, with the baggage on the roof, where I have an open view of the passing rice fields and mountains. A noticeably well-nourished Filipino clings fast to a spare tire next to me. His perfect English gives evidence that he doesn't belong among the poor: Harry is studying law, will soon take his State exams, and is presently on his way back to Manila. As I explain to him that I'm from Switzerland, but live in Bagong Silang, he shakes his head: "Impossible. No Europeans live there." Then he idly lights a new cigarette with the glow at the end of the one he just finished. Somewhat self-importantly he explains to me that he knows the slums and settlements from his volunteer activities, providing help to the poor regarding their rights.

"Come visit me," I try ending the conversation. His type no doubt belongs to the well-nourished Filipinos who glibly like to pretend to do something for the poor. He wants to know my exact address. It's all for show; he's really not interested. Beyond that, he adds that he's in the process, with other departing students, of founding a non-governmental organization (NGO) in order to provide a framework for their lawyerly volunteer work.

I am positively amazed as this Harry Roque and his fellow student, Joel Butuyan, appear at the "Orphanage" a few days later. His red car in the midst of the impoverished shacks is truly an alien object. They have put up with two hours of exasperating driving through the city to get here. How wrong one can be about people! As I see both of the prospective lawyers sitting on the floor with our boys, chatting and eating, I get the happy impression that Harry and Joel will be back. The encounter on the Jeepney roof will yet have a meaningful sequel.

James, the Trades Union Steward

Outside, in front of my shack, a few of my bodyguards huddle and learn to read and write. Albert is their teacher—again someone whom I met on a language walk-about. The approximately thirty-year-old man sports a tattoo of a cannabis leaf on his upper arm, and the mark of a somewhat notorious gang on his back. During a knife fight, Albert lost his leg and for some years now, he's had a wooden prosthesis. In prison he began to pray, and with the help of an American missionary found a position as a caretaker in a theological institute, where he learned English—and read the Bible.

When I met him, he was a kind of freelance, self-proclaimed evangelist without a regular income, who, with his aged mother, barely managed to survive. After I watched Albert for a few days and spoke to him several times, I asked if I could employ him as a teacher for my ever greater number of bodyguards. He

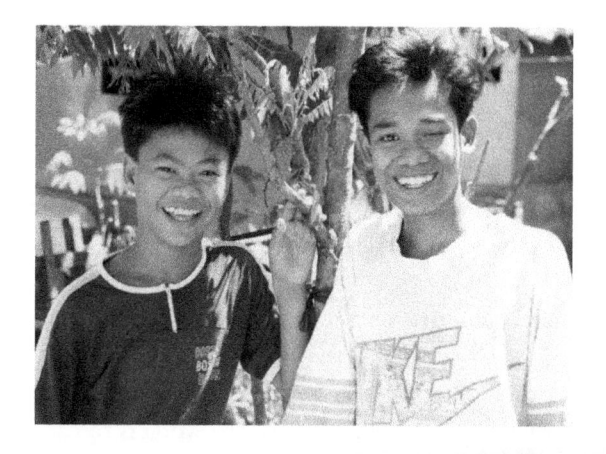

Always right in the picture: Mata, with and without his eye!

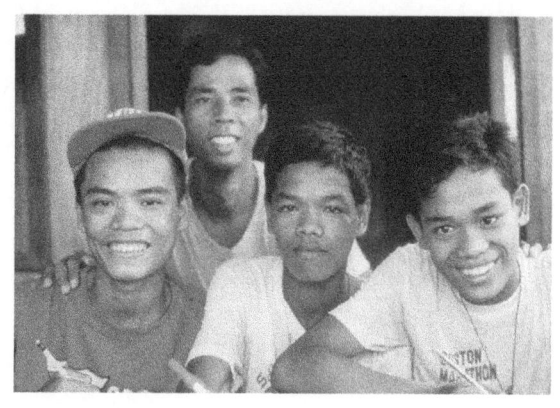

The neglected boys, my bodyguards, learn to read and write with Albert (in the background)

was pleased and beamed, like a little boy. And now he sits in front of my hut and instructs the boys in reading and writing.

One of the most avid students is Mata. I am really proud of the boy. I explained to him that the man on the crucifixes that are found everywhere around here, rose from the dead, and that he wants to give him the gift of life as well. This apparently clicked with him. "Jesus is now my friend," he says, and blossoms and grows with a joyful demeanor.

I wish I could acquire a glass eye for him. He suffers quite a lot because of his missing eyeball and the ugly wound. Filipinos know they are attractive, and value their appearance. Many make a great effort to take good care of themselves, even and especially here in the slum.

My work is significant: The boys progress; I progress. Our friendship enlivens us. Sometimes the initiative to read the Bible actually comes from the boys. Individuals often react to the stories about Jesus of Nazareth with intense emotional outbursts. Hearing about unconditional love exceeds their ability to comprehend. When, once again, their hard shells break open on one of these evenings in front of the shack, I wonder how it is that this Jesus of Nazareth has captivated people to such an extent for 2,000 years.

The friendship with James, on whose parcel my house stands, inspires me. He is only a little younger than I am, also single, lives next door, and speaks pretty good English, which is very helpful to me in my interaction with the boys. James was always among the best in his class when he was a child and made it to the university, where he studied criminology. He had to leave after the first half year because his family ran out of money. For years he worked in a factory, completely below his capabilities, yet without prospects for advancement. Instead, he founded and led a workers' union.

"Do you know why I became a Marxist?" he once asked me, and immediately offered the impassioned answer himself. "Because the workers toil and toil, and still it's not enough. I've seen so much! Once I saw how the company doctor in a rubber factory falsified the protocols of the obligatory health checks of the workers, including X-rays, because these exploiters would have had to improve the working conditions, which was too expensive."

James's career as a Marxist trades-union leader came to an end when he was attacked one night by a hired gang. With a head fracture, he lay unconscious for hours in the gutter. Since then, James had to give up his factory job and live at home, unfortunately beset with regular headaches. An exception occurs when the boys and I sit in front of the shack in the evening. Then he often joins us, and listens attentively. Often the two of us have discussions, sometimes for hours, in English. He particularly admires the God who stands on the side of the oppressed. The places in the Gospel of Luke, where the expected Messiah purges the proud from the throne, and forces the rich to leave empty handed, or the passages from the Epistle of James about the cry of the exploited workers, whom God hears and for whom he becomes Judge and Avenger—they speak to his heart.

A few days ago James told me that for the first time in his life he felt peace in his heart. That made me intensely happy. The impassioned love for one's neighbor seems to me to be far more socially radical than class war.

I have a somewhat different friendship with Glenn Miles. He is a professional caregiver and student of theology from England who visited me for a few weeks. Determined to improve the world, he arrived in Bagong Silang with a certain naiveté, as most do. After Glenn once watched Mata stand in front of the mirror in the shack for a very long time and sadly study the hole in his face, he offered to go to the city to the eye specialist or to the social service office with Mata.

"Okay, go ahead," I told him—and silently I thought: You will have an interesting experience with the "social services" of Manila.

When I speak with Glenn, I notice that I have learned some things in the last half year, and that I not only live in Bagong Silang, but have also assimilated.

Imprinted Images

Ruth wrote me a letter a few days ago, saying that she admires me. Next to me, she feels like a worm, she said. "That embarrasses me," I answered, "the worm is namely me, and sometimes I ask myself what actually keeps me here. Maybe the Swiss sense of duty that I was raised with? Or maybe it's God's grace?"

One thing is certain: I have to find a path to an intimate relationship with Jesus of Nazareth again—otherwise this work will consume me. Physically, I feel well, except for my stomach, which gives me problems again and again.

Last night, a little two-year-old child died nearby. He had a fever for a whole week and received no medical care. We first heard about him when it was already too late. These are the unbearable moments....

As is customary, when someone dies in the immediate vicinity, I visit the family. Glenn accompanies me. The child's little corpse lies on a makeshift bier in a wretched shack. The mother is inconsolable. As we pray with her, I discover in the semi-darkness the little sister of the deceased boy. She is completely emaciated and seems feverish. Suddenly, she vomits and I am overwhelmed with horror: It is a large ball of long, live worms, thicker and longer than earthworms. We don't have any medications or remedies with us, but promise to return the next day and to decide then how we can help. On the way home, the image of that girl is indelibly etched in my mind. Despite a certain familiarity with misery, again and again there are certain impressions that make me shudder violently.

In the evening, a cool breeze blows, and the weather is right for letter writing. I would like to set up a kind of sponsorship program with my friends in Switzerland. Besides "my" boys whom Albert teaches, there are approximately thirty children and teens in the neighborhood who don't have the means to attend public school. They *must* get help! But then a mother appears, towing her howling eight-year-old son. She apologizes several times for the interruption. The boy has had stomach pains for a number of days, she says. I carefully feel around the stomach area. The appendix is either severely inflamed or has already burst. Frenziedly, we arrange transportation to the hospital, and again I feel this rage rise in me. One hundred forty thousand residents and no hospital for them!

On another morning, I allow myself an extended jog. I have finally found a good route. At least when I'm jogging, I'm alone with God and with myself. Thoughts and ideas come up that transcend the activities of the day and propel me to keep going. Sometimes, doubts run along with me, wondering whether this all makes sense or if it's only mere activism. Two hours later I'm back in our little clinic and don't have time for doubt any longer.

In the evening on my way home, I see Mata sitting in front of our shack. The boy spots me, leaps up, dashes towards me, and bubbles over with a flood of Tagalog. Glenn steps out of the hut and tells me that they both were at the Makati Medical Center. Typical of Glenn, I think, marching directly into the most renowned and most expensive hospital in all of Manila. Apparently he had success.

"We traversed the corridors until we found the Chief of the Eye Clinic, an old professor in an elegant, air conditioned office. I believe he found us a somewhat remarkable twosome, I as a Brit, and Mata. In any case, he listened to us attentively, and then he thought for a short while and said: "In ten days I am going to retire. I will personally make a glass eye for you. Let the cost be my problem." Glenn grins.

A short time thereafter James returns home, completely upset. I ask him what happened. We sit down in front of his small house and he says: "Finally, at long last, I once again was able to fight my way into the seat next to the Jeepney driver today—of all days. In front of the factory near Novaliches where I was once employed, workers on strike stood across from a group of security officers, and we couldn't get by. The workers started to throw stones. And then the security forces opened fire. They shot directly at the workers! Our driver wanted to get out of the line of fire, but we couldn't back up because there was a traffic jam behind us. So he simply stepped on the gas and tried to escape by going forward. The women in the Jeepney screamed like crazy. I saw many people who had been shot, and I recognized three of them as we passed nearby. They were innocent factory laborers!"

Later we're sitting with the teenagers but James seems very distant. One senses how the old scars of the former fighter in the battles of class conflict have re-opened. Even "peace in one's heart" is fragile here.

Snake Island

Mata laughs. The old professor actually did make him a glass eye—and what an eye! It sits so perfectly in the eye socket that he can actually move it a little with the remaining muscle, and is so deceptively real that only with difficulty can one distinguish it from Mata's natural eye.

"Now that you're no longer one-eyed, the name Mata doesn't apply any longer," I say. Unanimously the teenagers determine to call him by his real name, and Mata becomes Brian. He beams. I gladly welcome this image to be indelibly burned into my mind.

Ralph and Irene Dörpfeld from Switzerland come for a visit. Together with Volker Heitz, Ralph is the pastor of my Christian Fellowship at home, the Evangelical Community Basel (EGB). They'll be here approximately two or three weeks. Ralph has determined that he wants to found a branch of Servants in Switzerland. It is absolutely grand how completely the EGB stands behind me and how the faithful are interested in, and support, my work here.

On another day we set out for our little weekend camp at Snake Island in the Bay of Olongapo—in addition to me, there were about two dozen kids including a couple of girls, as well as Pepe Jose Gonzales, an enthusiastic young pastor about my age. The kids are euphoric, and we're happy too. At last, a respite from the dregs!

The trip to Snake Island takes a number of hours and is tortuous. The Jeepneys have no springs and are far too low for a European. After ten minutes, my neck and the small of my back already hurt. The road dust burns my eyes, the diesel fumes burn my nose. At the coast we buy several plastic containers of drinking water, climb into the ferry-boat, and cast off.

As we approach the island, I become disillusioned: Although there are coconut palms and shrubbery, the beach is full of accumulated trash, and the water is murky. A million mosquitoes welcome us. The girls and boys hardly seem to notice. They happily carry the water to a shady place and put the little tents together with the plastic flats. In addition, we walk along the beach around the perimeter of the island. During a short swim I make the acquaintance of a few jellyfish whose long filaments burn my skin like fire ants.

Towards evening we cook rice on an open fire. The kids are more joyful than ever. They must have the opportunity to escape Bagong Silang far more often. After the meal we sit in a circle and sing songs into the night. Pepe knows the songs and takes the lead, and the children repeat the words, more or less in tune. Pepe's enthusiasm and capability are infectious, and he knows Tagalog besides. . . .

I have prepared a Bible text, from the second chapter of the Epistles of St. Peter, not only as input for the kids, but also as a language lesson for myself. So I sit down and tell these young, dispossessed slum dwellers, these nobodies without possibilities, that they are living stones with which God is building a house so that he can live within them: "Each of you counts, each is important, each is worthwhile."

Suddenly one begins to cry loudly. I pause for a moment. Another one starts. A half minute later almost all the boys and girls are crying, loudly and without restraint. This is totally unexpected. Pepe looks at me. We are quiet for a long moment, to allow the episode to run its course. Some tremble, a few others kneel down. It seems as if a dam has been broken and a mighty flood of pain, frustration, and misery flows forth. Pepe and I also begin to weep. Then we place our arms around the shoulders of one after another, pray, and bless them.

It takes a while for the flood to ebb. As I lie down, I've completely lost track of time. I can't fall asleep yet, in order to hold fast this holy, liberating moment just a little longer. God is present.

As we return from our little weekend camp, the island has taken on a new meaning for me, despite the trash and mosquitoes.

The Left Curve

I'll never be a fan of the Jeepneys, and even less of the Philippine potholes and the drivers who ride roughshod over the planks that cover them. Celso also drives in a spirited fashion, but in comparison to others here in the area, his style is bearable. We've been traveling over two hours and the atmosphere on board is good over all. In addition to five teens from the youth group and me, two interns from a Theological College from the UK, Vreni Anliker and Glenn Miles are also with us.

We're on a fact-finding mission which will include an overnight rest stop in the fresh air outside the city. We want to find an appropriate place for the next outdoor camp for the youth group. These little excursions are good for me, just as the regular respites at the Servants house. On these trips one's thoughts are also free to fly, and one sees certain things differently from a bird's-eye perspective. . . .

Since our camping trip to Snake Island much has transpired. The Swiss sponsorships for our students are secured. We can finance several teenagers' attendance at the State school, and others are taught by Albert. They are progressing more quickly in reading and writing than I am in Tagalog. In the meantime we have

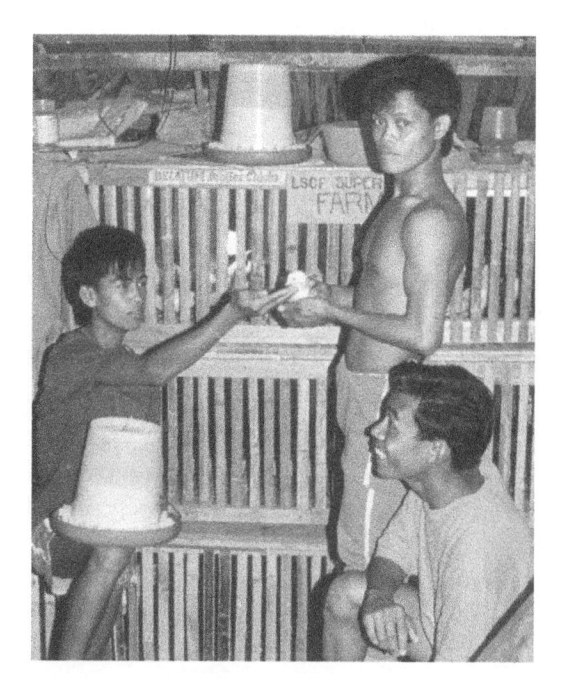

We built a small chicken-coop alongside our own little house. Now my bodyguards have some work and can help earn their meals. In the middle of the picture, Noriel.

built a pigsty for Albert next to his hut and have bought him several piglets, so that he need not depend on my salary payments. And adjacent to our own little house, we have built a little hen house. Now my bodyguards have some work and can earn their keep.

Our "Orphanage" is bursting its seams. I have forbidden the boys a number of times to bring new members into the youth group. Nonetheless, there are now about forty teenagers who meet three evenings per week. They come here with only one or two meals in their bellies, gather together and without encouragement begin to sing and to pray—as a group, these youths have developed an extraordinary dynamic.

There are so many that come now that I can't oversee each individual optimally. Consequently, I am not unhappy if I can place one of them elsewhere, such as Reymond. The fourteen-year-old with the beautiful face now and again played the high spirited young man, but mostly one sensed a certain restlessness in him. It turned out that he, with his gang, had demolished his own school house and now, with me, sought to hide from the police. I was not happy with this idea. Luckily, I could place him with a friend whom I knew from our regular retreats at the Servants house. He works in a distant inner-city slum, sufficiently far away from the local police.

It often gives me enormous pleasure when I can experience, along with them, how these youngsters are able to change. Nonetheless, I'm exhausted more often than I care to admit. The oversight and monitoring are far more important than I had imagined. The boys are compelled to switch back and forth between two worlds: Here the group with its familiar characteristics, there the usual context of their neighborhoods and relations. Old habits such as gambling or jealousy undermine the boys and disturb the social system. Sometimes it happens that the money for school is not spent for notebooks or uniforms, but rather disappears on the gambling table—their poverty spawns the hope that with a little luck more money can be made, and hope dies last. Then I, as the distributor of the sponsorship money, am told various embarrassing lies of necessity.

The sponsorship program is sometimes also sabotaged because of illness and hunger. Isn't it understandable that rice and milk or medications are sometimes more important than registration fees or the money for the Jeepney trip to the state school? Fortunately, in the supervision of the boys, I have the support of several reliable local colleagues. We are involved in their nutrition program and their medical aid. Relative to the general situation in Bagong Silang, our system functions reasonably well.

A good network is important to us. The people around Rob and Lorraine belong to the network as well as the other slum workers, as do European practitioners such as Glenn or Vreni, who now sit next to me and apparently feel as little affection for the lurching Jeepney and the erratic driving style of Celso as I do. . . .

The good mood of the boys is nonetheless infectious, and as they begin to sing loudly, my thoughts return to the happy anticipation of our little camp. We're close to the goal and need only a good place to erect the tents. The boys sing at the top of their lungs, Celso accompanies them happily with the Jeepney's horn, and veers into a left curve, and I instinctively sense that we're going too fast—we're going to go off the road.

A jolt—the right wheel has overshot the edge of the street. A violent shudder follows. "That's it," races through my mind, and I press down against the floor of the Jeepney. It rumbles and cracks, followed by a deafening grating of fracturing metal. Then suddenly, all is quiet.

First I'm numb. But then the odor of seeping diesel oil stings my nose. My adrenalin kicks in, so to speak, and in a second I am outside. The others, too, manage to crawl out of the wreck under their own power. The vehicle is upside down. Emer is crying hysterically for his Mama. Vreni smiles absentmindedly, walks a few steps, and collapses. I briefly provide first aid. Then I read the clearly defined tire marks and reconstruct the accident: We were careening toward a pole, Celso wrenched the steering wheel to avoid it, the Jeepney catapulted across the main street in the direction of a ravine, barely missed the concrete wall of a bridge, rolled over, and slid on its roof about ten yards over the asphalt, back to our side of the street, where it stopped at the sloping bank. Now I begin to quake from head to toe.

Hardly a half hour later the wounded are in the nearby district hospital. The accounting: Abrasions and bruises, a larger gash, and Vreni has a broken collarbone. It's hard to grasp: That's all. One feels as if one has been called back to life anew.

The days after the accident are more intense than usual: Colors, smells, sensations, feelings, people. Life is incredibly alive, and in everything I recognize the spirit of God. It is life as a gift. I am happy about everything and am grateful. I often think especially of my friends and relatives in Switzerland who, I know, are sharing and praying with us.

I often ask myself during these days what actually is important in life. In the face of one's own death, one's daily struggles pale. More than once I ask God for the ability to slow down in my new life, so that I don't lose track of his voice in the midst of my own activities. I especially seek to preserve the nearness of God during these days, to experience the small miracles as small miracles—to see, to hear, to smell, to sense the smile or the touch of another person, to enjoy a good conversation deep in my soul—or simply cool water on a hot day.

Reymond, the Teenager

Reymond has returned. He became too bored at my friend's in the inner-city slum. The police arrested him and stuck him in a cell, beat him up, and threatened him with "salvaging," the peculiar name they give to their brand of mob law. After a few days they released him. Now he's showing up here a lot. Of course, he can't go to school any longer, and except for his overly burdened mother, the unruly teenager apparently is completely alone.

Since our "Orphanage" was founded six months ago, many teenagers have advanced through a good deal of development. Reymond, however, seems stalled. He often appears to be sad and preoccupied, and avoids direct eye contact at all times. Since I've become able, in the meantime, to engage in simple conversations with my translators, I seize the opportunity at one point when we're alone and ask: "Rey, what's going on with you?"

Rey ponders a while, and then he answers: "I hate myself. I can't stand myself any longer."

"I take it that you have a reason."

Rey says nothing.

"You are very worthwhile, and I like you very much, Rey, but even more important, God loves you."

"I hate myself because I'm so bad."

"What makes you so bad?" I probe carefully.

Rey hesitates again, and then says abruptly, "A girl wanted to join our gang. She was young and a virgin. We asked her, 'How do you want to pay your entry fee, with a beating or with love?' Then we all raped her—one after the other."

A deafening silence follows. I've heard some weighty confessions in the past, but this one almost took my breath away. Not only because in the Philippines rape is punished by death,* but above all because of the burden on Rey's soul.

"I can never again be happy like you," Rey says and begins to weep.

---

* The death penalty in the Philippines was abolished by the late president, Gloria Arroyo, in 2006.

It must be horrible to have to live with such a deed and to know that nothing can ever undo it. Here is this good-looking boy with his large child-like eyes, and such a drama rages in his heart. I pray for the right words and a miracle.

"A radical solution is the only answer for you," I say cautiously. You need a new heart, so that you can slowly become new again, from within." A long conversation follows, about the punishment for transgressions and about the God who became man. "Jesus of Nazareth hung your guilt up on the cross," I say to him, and then we pray.

Just days later, we suffer a severe blow. Rob and Lorraine have gone home to Australia, probably forever. For some time now they seemed tired and lacking in strength. Just a short time ago I read an article about a new sort of societal illness, "Burnout Syndrome." Now I know what is meant by that. First the heart is inflamed about something, and then it burns out. The departure of Rob and Lorraine is very much on my mind during these days, even though the clinic, the boys, the sponsorship program, and everything else keeps me on the run. And without mentioning that after Rob's return home, there are people who expect that I'll become pastor of the orphaned Living Spring Fellowship. Well, great. . . .

Shortly thereafter Mike, my team leader whom I see from time to time at the Servants house, visits us in Bagong Silang. The New Zealander lives with his family of four at the edge of a river in a wretched, miserable slum with approximately 10,000 residents. There he serves as the pastor of a Christian community which he founded—no small task. Mike is the only one on the Servants team who keeps current by reading the professional literature and by writing articles about community development in urban poor settings.

Normally Mike is very conscientious and disciplined. But as he looks at our work, his expression noticeably darkens. Later, as we sit in front of my little hut, his collar bursts: "We are all beginners in this development work," he scolds, "but you are the worst of all! You've gotten ahead of yourself in every way! First comes the language and the deeper understanding of the culture here . . . of the culture of poverty and the Filipino culture. Only then can you wade in! But you dove in so quickly that you'll make mistakes that won't be able to be undone!"

My attempts at justification fail miserably. Mike cannot be persuaded, and—he is right. Instead of entirely devoting myself to the language and culture in this first year, I am almost completely and exclusively involved in projects. I've started a support program, founded a youth group, organized a leisure-time activities scheme for teenagers; I bear the responsibility for an emergency clinic,

I allowed water fountains to be drilled and initiated, together with Rob, the founding of neighborhood organizations. I've been active in job-generating projects and, in just a few weeks, my living quarters transformed themselves into an "Orphanage."

After Mike handed me my head, we're both similarly depressed. I'm obliged to believe him. He is responsible for an international team of daring novices. As do all of us, Mike also lives mostly at the borderline of his limits. Just a couple of weeks ago, he lost his own child. His brave wife, Rubi, had become infected with a virus during her pregnancy and Joseph was born too soon, too weak to survive more than a few days.

We're silent for a while. Then Mike says, "You have to leave Bagong Silang, and quickly. Find a settlement in the city where the need is not as overwhelming as here."

I ask myself if Mike blames himself that now, after four years, Rob and Lorraine had to throw in the towel. They were his pioneering friends from the first hour forward. He surely wants to prevent the same thing from happening to me. Mike is right, and I know it. I have to start again, from the beginning.

Moving to Bagong Barrio

My new start takes place in Bagong Barrio. The residential settlement—north of Manila, near the city beltway—is a former slum colony on government land. Some years ago the authorities promised to sell the occupied land to the settlers. Therefore the residents have improved their shacks, which are now solid, multi-story houses. Most of them are very narrow; almost nothing is planned and much is improvised, but nonetheless at least the wastewater canals are covered. There is running water; a few people even have a telephone. The district is described as a "semi-depressed area" and consequently occupies a higher step in the social hierarchy than an illegal slum, whose residents are constantly threatened by eviction.

As a result of my move, I have more or less ascended—to a room of raw cement bricks with a cement floor and a corrugated metal roof. It sounds stable, but everything is somehow lacking in density, with inferior plaster work. Rainwater runs through the cracks in small rivulets.

What disturbs me more are the rats and giant cockroaches that build their nests in the many dirty, damp joints and apparently feel comfortable there. Above all, they come out at night and throw merry parties, with a lot of movement and noise. A mosquito net protects me from the disgusting cockroaches, but there doesn't appear to be a remedy against the rats. Again and again, I wake up and can't get back to sleep because of the squeaking and rustling. Once, I spring up in fright—right next to my head a gigantic rat squeaks in the semi-darkness.

I feel the anger rising, raise my fist, and strike out with all my might. Of course the rat is quicker, and my fist thunders into the unpolished cement wall. My skin is shaved off, the bones in my hand are exposed, it hurts horribly and bleeds, and the mosquito net has been ripped and pulled down. I am a complete idiot.

I don't have a toilet. My landlord and his family live next door and have invited me to use theirs. That's fine and during the day quite practical. However, if I have to go at night I find their door locked. The children lie like sardines on the floor behind the door and sleep.

My worst toilet problem, however, once occurred on the road. Together with a friend I am riding in an old Jeep that belongs to Servants on the Harbor Road that leads to Navotas, where we want to visit a project. The Harbor Road runs along a mile-long settlement that was once known by the legendary name, "Tondo," as the largest slum in Asia. Suddenly I have an acute problem, namely stomach cramps, that announce impending diarrhea. Wouldn't you know, right here and now....

"I have to get out, urgently and immediately, otherwise I'll explode," I call out to my companion. At first, he grins. But then he sees my panicked expression and understands. We promptly drive to the nearest slum shacks and ask for a toilet. "Sorry, Sir, we don't have a toilet here ourselves."—"Okay, quick. Let's go," I moan. I imagine what would happen, if.... We are at least one hour by car in heavy traffic away from home and far and wide, not a tree, only people, cars, and shacks!

About a hundred yards farther we stop again: "We urgently need a toilet! Immediately, please, please!" The answer is the same: "Sorry, no toilet here, keep looking, maybe farther up the road or over there." This can't be real! Thousands of slum shacks in the middle of the city and not one with a toilet! It gives new meaning to the old concept of "pressing need." The trick with a newspaper comes to mind, the "roll-and-throw method": One takes an old newspaper, lays it on the ground and does one's business on it. Then one wraps the stinking pile carefully with the newspaper, puts it into a plastic bag, and throws the little package into the trash or into the river at the earliest opportunity—a humiliating experience that many of the poor experience on a daily basis.

But roll-and-throw is no longer a possibility; my intestine is about to explode. Again and again we try our luck in vain. I curse and pray and cramp and pray and curse, until I'm dizzy. Suddenly, my companion calls out: "A hut with a toilet!" I bolt inside. It's occupied!

I crumple down on the floor in front of the door of the toilet. In this position each second becomes an eternity. The door finally does open and I actually make it.... The word "timely" is out of place here after this agony. The aftermath is holding one's tongue; water, soap, gratitude, and a few *pesos* for my saviors—and, the realization, how little a person sometimes needs to be happy again.

The Freedom of a Motorcyclist

My concerted effort in Bagong Barrio again is learning Tagalog. In Jesse Sarol I find a very good private teacher who soon also becomes my friend. For the first time I have the feeling that I'm making forward strides in the language. Finally!

Naturally, despite the move, I have not become detached from Bagong Silang. I am now simply a commuter. In the meantime I actually have acquired my own vehicle—a motorcycle. Generally, private vehicles are not a part of our equipment, but the team granted me the purchase of a Honda in my second year. My Servants colleagues are consistent and really move about only on public transportation. To live with the poor means learning to live with the feeling of being on the side of the losers. And a loser does not ride a motorcycle.

Nonetheless I quiet my guilty conscience regarding this privilege because its practical use prevails. I oversee communities and projects in various areas of the metropolis, and I didn't come to Manila to spend my time waiting around, after all. Without a vehicle one stands distressingly long in the heat on dangerous curbs, waiting in vain for a bus or Jeepney. When one finally comes and with luck one has claimed a space, one stands squeezed between a mass of people, delivered up to the driving style of an overly tired driver, who agonizes his way through the traffic and speeds, and brakes, and honks without consideration. On the motorcycle I have the feeling of belonging to the winners, at least in the traffic of the urban metropolis. Speed, efficiency, and security: Advantages of the rich.

Many streets in Manila are often flooded up to a foot and a half after a heavy tropical rain. With my Honda, whose tailpipe is mounted just under the seat, I tack like a boat through the floods, past the stranded pedestrians—except last week, when I sank into an open wastewater canal together with the Honda, since missing canal covers and ditches are naturally not obvious in the dirty brew. But I got away relatively lightly with abrasions and contusions on both thighs and on my chest. And, in the meantime, I have the Honda back again, too.

Now and again I ask myself if the move was really sensible. At the very least, I live in Bagong Silang as much as I live in Bagong Barrio. The communities, the kids ... Reymond makes me especially happy when we regularly see each other in the Bible group. It seems as if he has really acquired a "new heart." He has become a reliable friend in the community, for whom nothing is too much. As I mounted the Honda today after our conversation-hour, he stood there and looked me in the eye, and laughed merrily. Hey, I enjoy that!

Back at home in Bagong Barrio, I first set up my newest acquisition: A rat trap. Originally, I wanted to start my campaign with rat poison, but the neighbors advised me against it. With poison in their bellies, the beasts hide in inconvenient places before they die. They rot there slowly and contaminate the entire house. Therefore I bought a rat trap at the market, a wire cage with a door that snaps closed. I set it up and went to bed.

The next morning one of the little monsters actually squeaks inside the trap. What do I do now? I ask a couple of the teenagers, who don't give me a real answer, but take the trap out of my hand and before I comprehend what they're doing, the cage—replete with contents—is soaked in gasoline and engulfed in flames. The rat squeaks, its burning flesh stinks, the boys laugh. My stomach almost turns over.

"It's very simple," Jesse tells me that afternoon. "You have to drown them. It's more humane, quick, and painless."

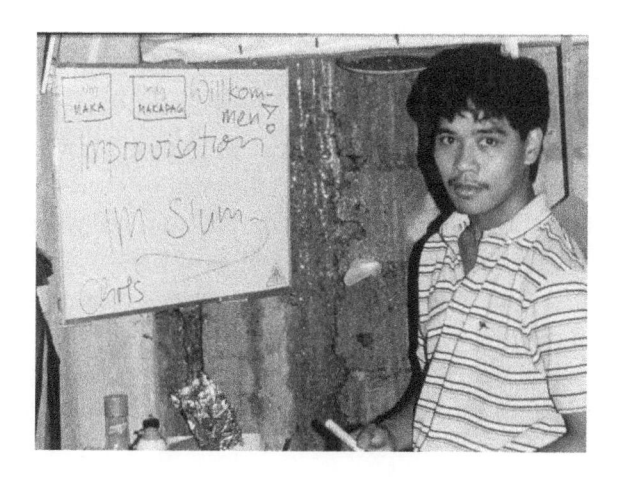

Language lessons with Jesse Sarol, in my new "rat-trap" in Bagong Barrio. One can see the rain running down the wall.

Two days later I once again have a rat in a cage, and I step up to the deed: Into the water. But the result is horrible; it seems to me as if the fight against death under water lasts an eternity. It's a nightmare. And the monster—that's me. As the rat finally gives up the ghost, I determine to do as millions of poor people have done, and live a kind of coexistence with the rats. If one kills rats, one neighbor tells me, then their companions will come in hordes; one mustn't begrudge one another a place to live. By all means. As far as I'm concerned, however, even if the rats are among God's creatures, they won't succeed in getting my sympathy.

I met Doc while jogging—a muscular guy, twenty-six-years-old, with a friendly face. Keeping up with him is completely impossible. Doc is a marathon runner and tries to achieve good rankings in competitive marathons, thereby winning a little cash from time to time. This is very welcome since his daily earnings are barely enough for food. For 56 *pesos*, approximately 2.5 US dollars, he cleans the toilets of a well known radio station six days a week, eight hours per day. This "wage" is a joke and represents not even half of the legally prescribed minimum wage.

Doc lives everywhere—wherever he can find accommodation: As an orphan from the provinces he has no relatives in the city. For the last nine months, the wooden bench in the office belonging to his boss has served as his bed. "This is better than a park bench," he explains to me, "the soot on the street makes me sick."

Doc does well. He is not as fatalistic as many others here; he searches for the small opportunities and grabs them. Perhaps to accomplish this, one simply needs the perseverance of a marathon runner.

The War

Normally, in the mornings even before the sun comes up, I go jogging. My new neighborhood is bounded on the east by a wall that is intended to sequester Araneta Park from the public. I found an opening in an inconspicuous place in this wall, and for weeks now I've been climbing through it every morning to jog on a thread of cement pavement between the trees. I thoroughly enjoy this more or less refreshing hour in the morning, when at least once during the day I can be alone with my thoughts and prayers, hear my own breathing, and at a good distance, the still tolerable noise of a city awakening.

The park is actually privately owned, but I don't have a guilty conscience. It is the size of eight soccer fields and borders a large slum on the east side, where the people live crowded together in dark shacks with just a few square feet at their disposal. From their perspective the immense park is simply a waste of space and a provocation at the same time.

As I awoke this morning, however, it immediately became clear that I wouldn't be jogging today. I could hear impassioned shouting from the street: "*Guierra na, guierra na!*" *war, war!* Is it war? I ask myself. As I got up, I could hear the noise of helicopters above the city and could make out muffled shelling far way. I quickly get dressed. As I step to the door, fighter planes thunder above, flying low over the houses. The noise is deafening. What is the reason for this? Over the following days we hang onto every word we hear on the radio or television, almost without interruption. A small group of army insurgents under the leadership of Gregorio Honasan have occupied parts of the business districts and exchange fire with troops loyal to the government of Corazon Aquino. The government troops, of course, have the upper hand. But officer Honasan is young and popular, and here in Bagong Barrio the people cross their fingers for the rebels. They cross their fingers for everyone who is against the government because they hope that finally something will change for the better.

It is an expression of despair: Until three years ago the dictator Ferdinand Marcos had ruled the land for twenty years, supported by the USA, until he allowed the leader of the opposition, Ninoy Aquino, to be murdered, thereby involuntarily inciting an uprising of the people and therefore having to flee the country. That was the famous EDSA Revolution. The insurrection swept Ninoy's widow, Corazon Aquino, to power, and all the hope of the opposition and the poor rested with her. Now, after three years only one thing remains: Bitterness.

We foreigners are instructed to stay indoors. I try to reach the Swiss Embassy by telephone but get no answer. Most of the skyscrapers in the business district where the embassies are also located are occupied by the rebels and are being shelled by the government troops. At the same time, in our part of the city, the days continue as if nothing were happening, with the exception of the live conversations on television about the war under way in the same city. How grotesque all this is!

The boys of Bagong Silang expect me to appear for our Bible-discussion Circle despite the events of the war. I ride there and it becomes a gripping afternoon. The actual events are completely engrossing, as we watch upsetting pictures of young Filipino combatants who, in these hours, are bleeding to death in the streets of Manila. Some of them are not much older than the boys present at the Bible Circle.

At this moment, all the existential questions that the Bible raises come to the fore once again. We too endure an ongoing battle. The young people here, constantly striving to survive and seeking to gain some advantage in this great sea of poor people, could also end their lives in death and defeat. Or they can pledge their life to the peaceable kingdom of God, to love and justice. They can resist evil, without violence, like Jesus. I sense an infectious joy and earnestness among the boys. We help one another in life to swim against the stream. As I climb back on my Honda, I feel stimulated and motivated.

Shortly before I get home, a car drives out of its parking place into the street without warning, and I end up in a heap. I'm catapulted against a dirty city wall. The driver of the car is a pleasant veterinarian who immediately takes me to his office behind the parking lot and pours pure alcohol on my abraded shoulder. I squeak like a pig before slaughter, but he seems unimpressed. Well, the man is, after all, an animal doctor. At least he is properly embarrassed, and he wants to know what has brought me, a Caucasian, to this part of Manila. Finally he promises me to come to Bagong Silang to teach our boys about how best to look after our chickens.

Nick, the Witness

In the middle of the night, someone knocks on my door. Nick stands outside, terrified. Sometime ago, at a Living Spring Fellowship service, he told me that he had been held captive in a cell by the police in Bagong Silang and under threat of death, set free. I ask him in, we sit down, and he tells me what has happened:

They, once again, carried out a police raid. Huts in disarray, a few boys led away in handcuffs, without a warrant. The angry parents came to me. I waited for Ronn in order to discuss how to proceed. You know I'm only the vice president, Ronn is the president of our self-help organization. Ronn immediately said that he would go forthwith to the police station. You've met him, too, a super guy, educated, with a good job, whom the police don't so easily put out of action.

I told him I would come later; I still had to eat something. Then I bought a little piece of roasted meat on a stick on the street and sauntered in the direction of the police station. There I leaned into the open doorway, chewing on my stick inconspicuously, and watched what was happening. Clearly, I was nervous. But,

I thought, maybe you'll learn something. Ronn has more experience in such situations than I do.

Ronn had made an effort to speak to the official in charge behind the desk. Men sat on hassocks and played cards. Many empty and half-empty beer bottles stood around. Actually, that's forbidden at a police station. Upon a signal from the duty officer, one of the men stood up and frisked Ronn for weapons from head to toe. He was obviously a police officer, in civilian dress; almost certainly, the other men around were also part of this police force.

Ronn stood quietly and allowed the examination of his body to take place. Suddenly, the man who was frisking him signaled his colleague. At first I thought that he had found something. The policeman shouted at Ronn, what was his problem! Ronn remained quiet, he didn't want to give them a chance to go on the offense. "Sir, I would like to know on what charge the boys from block 7 were arrested?" "That's none of your business," the police officer muttered. Quietly, Ronn said that he was the president of that neighborhood and represented the parents of the boys.

The officer shouted at him, that they were only doing their damn work, that it wasn't his business, and he should disappear. Then he pulled out his gun. I couldn't see if he shot intentionally, but the man was drunk. In any case, a shot rang out and hit Ronn in the upper thigh. He fell down and his wallet fell out of his jacket pocket, full of bank notes. Paper money fell on the floor and everyone present leaped up and grabbed the bills.

Then I saw, one of the civilians present lift a pistol in the air and yell: "Look, he's armed." He held the pistol wrapped in a towel and it became clear to me what was about to happen. "Ronn never had a weapon!" I shouted, and dashed into the room. Ronn lay in the middle of this chaos in a blood puddle. Apparently, the bullet had torn the artery in his thigh. He gasped and lost consciousness.

Naturally, the police locked me up. I still saw, however, how they heaved Ronn onto the cargo bridge of the police jeep. What a travesty! Later they tied me up and crammed a dark sack over my head, saying they would relieve me of my worries. Then they drove me around, and somewhere I had to get out and on my knees. They held the revolver to my head and pressed the trigger, without ammunition, again and again. I was terrified and they were amused by my fear. I didn't know if they were simply playing Russian roulette and would simply shoot me at the end. But afterwards, they drove back, let me out of the jeep, and told me I should disappear from Bagong Silang. They would murder me if I ever told anyone what happened at the Police Station.

Nick was trembling and my heart was pounding. I told him, he could of course stay with me, and Nick accepted my offer gratefully.

The next morning I went jogging again, except not in the park. The watchman had caught me a number of times and was less and less pleasant each time. The park belongs to the Araneta clan. This family is of Spanish descent, a large land holder, settled here since Colonial times. On Monday, the guard had finally threatened me with the police. That is too risky for me now.

But I have found a fine alternative for Araneta Park—a generously planted cemetery for the rich. I have to earn my restorative time between the graves daily with a quarter hour of all out running through quite dirty streets, a slalom through the morning dew, past gawking people, yelping mongrels, and stinking piles of trash. I'm not the only one, however, who enjoys the cemetery as the site of morning fitness training. I have made the acquaintance of other early morning risers. The cemetery is good for us. There are trees between the graves, the English lawn is beautifully groomed. The rich live better than the poor—even when they're dead. . . .

During the days, I again visit projects in Bagong Silang. At times riding my Honda I ask myself the question if the move to Bagong Barrio was actually necessary? I'm not only more deeply mired in the work of the projects, but in addition, also in the traffic. Not to mention that besides, I had fewer rats in Bagong Silang.

I bid my people in Bagong Silang goodbye in the evening. As I swing myself onto the Honda and head in the direction of Bagong Barrio, an old woman suddenly runs in my direction and shrieks like crazy. Somebody whispers: "Be careful, that is a witch!" To me, she seems disturbed, as she gesticulates wildly and pours curses and maledictions over me.

After a few minutes a dog runs onto the road, directly in front of my motorcycle. I avoid a collision only with great effort. With a pounding heart I keep driving. Twenty minutes later, a small child runs in front of the motorcycle. I brake hard, and begin to skid, but can maintain my motorcycle on its path. After a short, fervent prayer for protection I drive very carefully in the direction of Bagong Barrio. I'm not clear if this is just my overwrought imagination, or the "magical thinking" that leads to self-fulfilling prophesies. Perhaps the answer is far simpler, and the old woman is really a witch who can have an effect with her curses.

Two hours after my arrival, it's already dark, and Nick comes in. He is stressed. Despite his fear of the police he furtively went to Ronn's house and learned from his wife that Ronn is dead, due to loss of blood from the wound in his thigh. In short, he offered Ronn's wife his appearance in court as a witness if she were to bring charges against the police. Under these circumstances she is considering this, says Nick, and she knows an attorney. Certainly friends from the Living Spring Fellowship would also come to the proceedings and give her and Nick cover. Nick now knows, too, where the stuffed wallet in Ronn's jacket came from: It was Ronn's monthly salary and his Christmas bonus that he wanted to bring home from work that day.

Moving to Potrero

I've had enough of my rat hole without a toilet in Bagong Barrio. I've been here six months already, and that's plenty! I take off in the direction of Potrero—I want to get back behind the wall. It's peculiar, actually, that I had more rats in Bagong Barrio than in Bagong Silang.

Potrero is again a genuine slum, nothing about it is "semi-depressed." It's a pileup of intermingled, stacked plywood huts with corrugated tin roofs, through the middle of which a long column of cars that seems never to want to quit snakes its way. Not that the poor have cars here, but when the city highway traffic jams, then one can get to northwest Manila much faster by taking this narrow street riddled with potholes. And the highway is almost always jammed. Therefore, the slum dwellers use this needle-eye opportunity to fleece a kind of road toll from the drivers by way of collection boxes. One can consider this as a kind of compensation for the noise, the emission gases, and the street dust, which covers the people and their homes with a thick layer of dirt.

Within less than ten minutes I'm surrounded by a cluster of people. When I say that I'm looking for a place to live, general merriment breaks out. They suggest Araneta Village to me, on the other side of the park, since "people like you live there."

"No," I say, "I want to live with you." This produces only laughter, head shaking, and a surge of voices. A few days later, I try again. Maybe a few notice that I'm serious?

"I'm looking for a room, it can be very small," I assure those that are standing around. Again, head shaking and shoulder shrugs. Then suddenly I hear someone calling out of a dark alley, "Hey, Joe, come up here. Ate Donita wants to talk to you." Unknown Amerikanos in general are called Joe around here.

Two youngsters lead me a few steps along a dark path overrun with waste water, to a rickety staircase and up six feet to the first floor. It smells mightily of people, decay, and waste water. Nonetheless, I'm happily excited. At the door a middle-aged woman stands and smiles, and invites me in. This is apparently Ate Donita.

After the usual flowery phrases of greeting in astoundingly good English, she explains, "The house belongs to Lola (Grandmother) Lucia, my mother, and Papa Dela Cruz, my father. Although we live here in the slum, we are the rightful owners of this land and this house." This is very unusual.

I look around: The house is larger than usual, but quite run down. The *Sala* also serves as kitchen and bedroom for a part of the greater family. It's chock-full of plush animals packed in plastic and other kitschy memorabilia. To catch the eye, a giant color television stands in the middle of the room, naturally running without interruption, as with many of the poor—a small window into the world of the rich. I search in vain for the usually present house altar with figures of saints, candles or food offerings.

Ate Donita delivers a torrent of words. In the shortest time, she has explained the entire situation to me: She could install small walls for me with some plywood, that is, around the old, heavy Majong game table, since they didn't need the space or the table because they didn't want to earn money because of the neighbors' urge to gamble any longer, since they had become believers through Bible study at the home of a friend, where they had prayed for the healing of Lola Lucia, who was seriously ill with a hole in her spine from which fluid seeped constantly, but Lola Lucia recovered, upon which everyone entrusted themselves to this Jesus of the Bible, all but the men, who earlier had revered the figures of saints like gods, but now had removed them from the house, she herself was an optician and had to provide for her children and parents, and besides Lola Lucia was a healer with supernatural powers, and in case I ever have health problems she could help me, and Papa Dela Cruz was at the time of Ferdinand Marcos a community president and has remained a sort of father figure for all the residents of Potrero to the present day, whom one consulted when one needed his advice and help. . . .

My new home is a good fifteen square feet in size. Between plywood walls and roof there is an opening of one and a half feet—good for ventilation, bad for privacy—since a family lives on the other side of each of three of the four walls.

The discarded gambling table becomes my desk and dining table. I also have an old cupboard, but no plank-bed. At night I stretch out my mosquito net and unroll my sleeping mat on the floor. The toilet is located under the rickety stairs and is occupied by a couple of thousand hairy giant roaches. But one doesn't want to be too particular, it's a toilet! It is always available, also functions as a shower, and now and again water actually comes out of the hose!

Didn't I also, on my first night in Bagong Silang, feel a remarkable certainty of having arrived at the right place?

Christmas Stories

Christmas! The Rebel threat has been over for just a few days. One-hundred eighty soldiers and civilians were killed, they say. Honasan and his people lay down their arms, and the government promised them amnesty. But they won't be the last "disturbances."

As if peace would prevail in this land. Power-hungry leaders always find enough volunteers among millions of poverty-stricken people who have nothing to lose. The present war, the guerilla war of the Marxist New People's Army, has been going on for thirty years. I wonder how Nardo is doing? And Jovelyn, whom he left to join the resistance?

Yesterday I came from Potrero to Bagong Silang, where I will spend the Christmas holidays. I really looked forward to doing so. "*Maligayang pasko*," old and new friends called out to me, "Merry Christmas." And now I'm sitting here at the festive Christmas service of the Living Spring Fellowship, and I don't feel the least bit like celebrating.

This morning a woman, crying, told me that her husband had left her, without leaving anything of his Christmas money for her and her seven children, and had gone to his second wife. Again, in the last few nights, three young men were murdered in the immediate vicinity, seemingly without cause. One was stabbed on a public street, another at home, in his sleep. The third is my friend Do-Dong, a young and friendly boy, who used to join our fellowship meetings. Now he lies on a bier in his family's shack. He was stoned to death by drug addicts, people say.

At the end of the service the congregants make offerings to help two families—the first is one whose hut burned down with all the possessions that they had been able to accumulate in the last years. The second family had their clothes stolen while they and their five children were at the chapel for morning prayers.

Although most of the congregants at the service live below the minimum standard themselves, the collection yields 250 *pesos*, approximately the equivalent of four days' pay of a simple laborer. The second family, whose father is unemployed, offers his entire share of the collection to the family with the hut that burned down—such deeds constitute Christmas. Thanks to the Swiss Missions account, I can contribute a "credit" for the material for a new roof.

I should seek out opportunities to personally report such events in Switzerland, not only because of the donations, but also to show that particularly in the saddest corners of the world, lasting values endure.

Despite desperate need, Living Springs in Bagong Silang is an unusually happy fellowship. Living Springs Christian Fellowship is part of a network of small indigenous congregations in Slum areas, in many cases initiated by Servants workers. It's been six months since the last foreign workers left the group, but a staunch core of believers has crystallized, slum dwellers who have taken on the responsibilities: Albert begins with an alphabet class for twelve adults. Lilibeth, a Filipino physician from a wealthy congregation in Manila, offers outpatient appointments. She is inundated.

As workers for Servants, we also celebrate Christmas, very traditionally with Christmas carols, Christmas stories, and unwrapping presents. Among our colleagues there are families with children. The Christmas meal consists of the classic Anglo-Saxon festival menu: dry turkey with remarkable bread and vegetable stuffing, dry potatoes with green peas and salad without dressing. For dessert there is a solid Christmas cake, an indefinable dark mass that the Anglo-Saxons curiously call pudding; only the sweet icing appeals to me. Everyone is extremely happy about the festive meal; only I think longingly of cream schnitzel with noodles or roasted Swiss potato cake with bacon and egg, sunny-side up. I don't let on, and try to join in the merriment. But suddenly we hear cries for help and weeping in front of our door. Somewhat impetuously, our team leader from New Zealand, Ian, runs outside and I follow.

Unexpectedly, we find ourselves in the middle of a street fight. Ian places himself in front of a young man who, with a large stone fragment, is beating a man lying on the ground, bleeding. Another one trains his revolver directly at us.

Ian screams at him: "Put your revolver down. Now. Put your weapon away, that's enough!" Slowly, the armed man turns and finally disappears between the shacks. I help a man with a stab wound in his stomach into a vehicle and we organize transportation to the hospital.

Later we have a long discussion about judgment, intuition, and responsibility in such risky situations—stark reality pushes the Christchild aside on this evening. Later in the night, as we pray together for a time, the message of peace of Jesus of Nazareth returns with a vengeance even in this sad corner of the world. We humans are the manger in which God was born, I once read. That strikes the mark.

On Wednesday I receive a letter from Switzerland. My mother writes that approximately two weeks ago she suddenly became fearful for me and felt the need to pray for me intensively. She mentioned the day and the time. I did the math: It was the afternoon with the witch and my "almost accident." I don't know if I should consider this a coincidence or not. I have an uneasy feeling... but I hold on fast to Christ.

The belief in the supernatural and spirits seems laughable only in the West. Here, however, the belief in spirits is present in all of the slums, whether in Bagong Silang, Bagong Barrio, or in the slum where I live, Potrero. My "slumber mother," Ate Donita, told me a few days ago that her son Jeffry and his wife Rosalie, who earn their livelihood as dancers in a nightclub, were on their way home at two o'clock in the morning and saw the "White Lady" (an evil spirit) in an alleyway in the slum.

"For me it's different now," Ate Donita says. "Since I became a Christian, I don't see or fear the demons any longer."

On December 29th, we take a day trip with about forty young boys from Bagong Silang. We drive to a river where we swim, sing, and play, tell one another stories about experiences with God, and fill our bellies—which feels good! For many young men from the wretched slum, when looking back such a day trip represents one of the greatest experiences of their youth—a year's ending as a kind of new beginning.

Ate Donita, the Supplicant

I've started off well in Potrero. The fact that I just left the hospital, where they sewed up a gaping wound on the back of my left hand, doesn't alter the circumstances. Emancipation is at fault. Namely, from the beginning in Ate Donita's household, it made me angry that the men in the house considered themselves above pitching in with the housework. The idealist in me would fall into a bad mood, and then I would try to act as an example, helping now and again. In truth, it also had to do with my showing gratitude for Ate Donita's hospitality; it's not easy accepting gifts from poor people.

My attempts at housekeeping failed miserably, however, because of sexism . . . not on the part of the men, but rather because of the mother Lola Lucia who, like a Fury, regularly grabbed the dishes out of my hands when I tried to wash them. Today at noon her thesis that doing dishes was not intended to be men's work was validated: I stuck my fingertips, with washcloth, into the bottom of a dirty drinking glass, forcing half my hand into the cheap beaker, which breaks, and the edge cuts the back of my hand. Lola Lucia's loud shrieking caused this to be the event of the day. They sewed up my wound in the hospital—and I will never again dare to go near the dirty dishes. One to nothing: Lola Lucia.

Ate Donita has invited me again and again to come to her Bible hour. She meets with friends on a regular basis in the little room next to my wooden partition. There they pray for their alcohol- and "shabu"/ crystal meth-addicted husbands, sons, brothers, and nephews,* and hope for a miracle. Ate Donita would also like to have men in her prayer group, but I find new excuses each time. With my language study and my projects, I'm fully occupied, and besides, I don't want to be taken in so completely by need as I was in the beginning in Bagong Silang. And I also don't know how one handles the wretchedness of alcohol- and drug-addiction on a practical level.

The people in Potrero have become accustomed to me. Above all, the children and young people are happy to listen to me, and always have time for a chat, for jokes, or to play with the Amerikano. Their laughter lights up my life. The work with the youngsters appeals to me; I like the kids.

I often take my language-walks-about near the "Monumento," a large memorial in a giant traffic circle at the northern end of the city highway EDSA. Hundreds of stands line the street there. Quite a few of the Potrero residents make their living as street vendors or itinerant peddlers—the street provides their clientele. The poorest among the marketers have no money for permits and set up illegally somewhere. Their presentation consists mostly of a plastic plank on the ground and a cardboard box with the goods. The illegals have fewer clients and therefore more time for my experiments in language practice.

When I ask them about their day's earnings, I regularly become angry: A great part of their meager revenue is taken by the police, as bribes. The police are also poorly compensated and need such "salary increases."

---

* Crystal methamphetamine is a synthetic drug of the amphetamine group and is often described as the "poor-man's cocaine" because it has a similar euphoric effect. It becomes addictive more quickly than any other drug. In the Philippines it is known as "shabu".

Yesterday I met a man who was just in the process of extorting money from the illegals. He addressed me in broken English, asking where I was from, and declaring himself to be a policeman. I explained myself and carefully asked him for his identification. He tore his T-shirt away from his beer belly, showed me the large caliber revolver in his waistband, and growled: "That's my ID."

Carefully I told him about policemen who enter houses by force without warrants, conduct brutal searches, and arrest children or carry off other youngsters without appropriate clearance. He answered: "No one respects us, therefore we have no respect for the people. We do our damned job, understand? I love this city, I love the bad elements, I love the corruption—it's all a part of it."

Such an encounter does one in. One asks oneself how law and order is supposed to be established in such a land. With a strict regime that holds people's rights in contempt? So much seems so hopeless.

Days later Nick appears, back from the first hearing about the shooting at the Police Station where Ronn was killed. He is bitterly disappointed: He was the only one who appeared at court; no one from the Living Spring Fellowship was present. Not even Ronn's widow came, for whom he had taken the risk to appear as chief witness. She was bribed by the police with 50,000 *pesos* (at that time approximately 2,000 US dollars) so that she would withdraw her complaint. For her this money was more important than life. And since the police was unable to capture Nick before the hearing in order to silence or kill him, they bribed the plaintiff. Looking at it from that perspective, with his courage Nick was able to get 50,000 *pesos* for Ronn's widow. Nonetheless, he would have preferred justice.

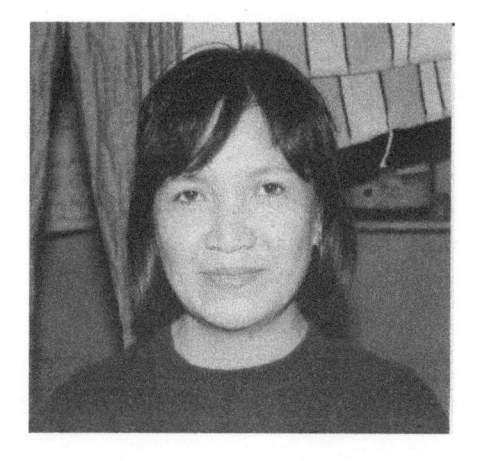

Ate Donita was the central person in the rousing of Potrero and is doing the same today in the new Community.

Nick says he's decided to find a place on the other side of the city. The risk of encountering the murderers from the police station there is smaller—a sad ending.

I, too, will have a new residence for a few months: From May until approximately October, I will be at home in Switzerland. There I will do one thing above all: Report, describe, explain—and plead for support, prayer, and engagement with the poor.

During this time I will be able to stay in a room in Riehen, in a large house belonging to the Schmidhauser family. Paul, the hearing- and sight-impaired father, and his wife and caregiver, Rosmarie, and the three teenagers, Andreas, Thomas, and Christoph, have grown close to my heart since the days of the Young Men's Christian Association. It's the Schmidhausers who are actually financing my journey. And before my trip to Switzerland, the Schmidhausers have allowed me to accompany them as guide, interpreter, and driver of their recreational vehicle along the east coast of Australia. They're giving me such a luxury vacation as a gift—me, a slum worker! It's overwhelming—and I'm so looking forward to it!

Reunion with Christine

What a green, clean, fresh, fragrant land! Not only is everything available in the supermarkets, one can have it in twenty varieties! Busses arrive on schedule; they don't drive—they float—straight ahead; seats are almost always available, and one hardly has to wait. On the street, I can understand everything that's said, even that which is none of my business. And I can get together with many friends, especially in my community, the EGB that supports me.

In this Swiss summer of 1990, I will: fourth, recharge; third, give lectures; second, co-found the Swiss branch of Servants; and first, enjoy relatives and friends. I was really looking forward to seeing them, and they were looking forward to seeing me.

Apropos of friends . . . Again and again in the last months I thought about Christine. I wondered if she'd come to hear one of my lectures.

In the meantime, Christine noted in her diary:

Typical. Christian Schneider is going to be on home leave in Basel half the summer long, and I will naturally be away at children's camps and youth group recreation meets during the same time. Oh, well, I'm not the only woman who is interested in this man anyway. But I can find out where and when he's going to lecture. Maybe I'll be lucky and one of the dates will coincide. One or two encounters will simply have to take place.

I feel an inner obligation to report to the people here about the ordeals of the slums. I cannot and do not want to remain silent about what I experienced. And certainly I'll be happy if, in describing my experiences, I succeed in having an effect on peoples' reactions—even if in the telling, an impression ensues that my life consists only of action and adventure. The reality of the many tedious days, between corrugated metal huts, where heat, air, and time stand still, and where desperation gnaws, is far less impressive than the reality of the misfortunes that I have encountered.

It's important that the people comprehend the gravity of the situation! We in the North have too much; they in the South have too little. We have the ability in our own hands to do something to change that. If only I could pull them out of their soft chairs and transport them to Potrero for an evening, so that they could also experience firsthand what goes on in my slums, while we sit here comfortably and shudder at my stories.

I passionately want to help people return to the actual meaning of being a Christian. We have to learn to read the Bible with new eyes. Then we might notice that words such as "poverty" or "poor" occur therein as often as the word "love." Actually I'm almost more of a missionary in Basel than in Manila—there for God, here for the poor.

I prepared most intensively for my course about "Mission and Social Responsibility," which I am offering at the Martin Luther King House in Basel. Here I can represent the values that are important to me and tell my listeners much about what I experience and understand in my "other life."

Among the participants I indeed discover Christine Tanner. She seems far less cool and distant to me than in those earlier days, when my brother Erich courted her in vain. She is six years younger than I am, so she must be twenty-five at this point. Her conversation is intelligent and engaged. It's astounding that such an attractive and busy woman has such an interest in the poor and weak of the world. And her blue eyes seem even bluer than before. . . .

Christine wrote in her diary:

I am inspired and touched by Christian's views of God and the world. It is exactly how I imagine a "mission": To live and suffer with the poor, instead of undertaking interventions into the world of the impoverished from the safe distance of a wealthy community. Would such a life in the slums of Manila be for me? Perhaps even together with Christian? Based on his glances and gestures, I have to conclude that he is not indifferent to me.

I am particularly happy that I visited my brother Erich. He works in Reichelsheim in Odenwald, where he has already been living for a few years, restoring a Gothic chapel and parts of a castle. In the meantime, he has become a competent master carver of stone. With his family he belongs to a vibrant ecumenical fellowship of families and singles named "Reichelsheim fellowship" (OJC: www.ojc.de); it belongs to the Evangelical Church in Germany (EKD) and maintains a protestant tradition inspired by Dietrich Bonhoeffer and Frank Buchmann among others. The community also supports my work in Manila. These are two weighty reasons for a visit to Reichelsheim.

It is good to see Erich; I enjoy the conversation between us brothers. We should do it more often! When I tell Erich that Christine Tanner attended my course in Basel, he says without hesitation: "She is an exceptional woman. And in case you have the slightest chance to marry her, take it."

Based on his glances and gestures, I have to conclude that he is not indifferent to me—that is laughable. Alright, down from the cloud. This man is one of those who have a friendly word for everyone, men and women. And also for me. What am I doing, counting on great possibilities here.

Erich leads me into the Knights' Hall of the castle and shows me a carving, which he shaped beautifully within a red sandstone column: A fox that stands upright and tries in vain to reach the abundance of grapes on the vine that hangs above him. "That's me," says Erich. He has carved his personal story here. For a long time, he has been working on other works of art, not the least of which is his family, together with his wife, Anne. A magnificent sculptor with passion, my "little" brother!

In the next weeks, I ponder Erich's words more than once. I'm not exactly on a bride-seeking path. Several short friendships, all of which I ended myself, are behind me. I believe that at age thirty-one, I have somehow imagined my life as one of a bachelor.

In the same week I visit the office of Horst-Klaus Hofmann, the founder and leader of the OJC. He is an author and widely traveled lecturer with a full calendar of appointments. I feel flattered. Purposefully and with probing glance, he poses the most extraordinarily personal questions.

"Which financial needs in Manila are the most pressing?" he finally asks.

"We have enough support for the projects under way," I answer. "But there is this project for legal help for the poor, a new initiative by my friends Harry Roque and Joel Butuyan. With 30,000 Swiss francs, these young lawyers could provide more targeted assistance to the residents of the slums who have no resources. In some cases, innocent youths sit in prison; in others, residential-, property-, and human-rights are transgressed." I hit my stride. "And you know what? The Christian communities don't want to give me any money for this!"

Horst-Klaus hits the table with his bare hand: "Well, come now! As if the rights of the poor are not a mandate from the Bible?! We will help you with this. All that I need is a written proposal." Wow, that sounds great! And I suspect that this could be the beginning of a longer partnership with the OJC.

At the University of Basel I give a lecture about the misery in the megacities of the Third World and the growth of the slums. One of the students stands up and makes a recommendation regarding how one might be able to halt people from abandoning the countryside: "A project is needed which will motivate and support the families from the slums to return to the provinces and build an alternative community there, combined with an agricultural project, that together would serve as a model so that others will follow this example." The idea fascinates me.

On July 16, a Monday, I sit with the Schmidhauser family in the kitchen, having supper. The radio plays in the background. "A violent earthquake has shaken the Philippines today." I hold my breath. "According to seismological reports, the strength of the quake was measured as 7.8 on the Richter scale."—*7.8, Oh dear God!*—"The epicenter lay northwest of the capital, Manila. According to the first estimates there are several hundred dead and thousands are injured. Experts expect an increase in the number of victims, since many people are still missing."

My heart begins to race. "Northwest of the capital, Manila" can mean a lot of things. Depending on the distance, "my" slums can also be affected. And I'm sitting here in Switzerland. A telephone call later, I know that Manila has barely noticed the quake. Instead, heavily damaged is Baguio City, which is the "summer capital" in the mountains of the Benguet Province north of the main island Luzon, on which Manila is located. The Philippines, sadly, hold the world record for tornadoes, floods, volcano eruptions, and other natural catastrophes. Why does it always happen to the poor?

What is going on with me that again and again I think about Christian Schneider; that the longer I lie awake, the more I ask myself whether a life in a slum would be a possibility for me. The area of Little Basel is no slum, but because of its large population of foreigners, some call it "Little Istanbul." That I work as a teacher of foreign-speaking children, and moved here two years ago in order be closer to the culture of this group and these children, is also a kind of mission.

The life here appeals to me: joyful, loud, colorful, and natural, also less orderly than in other quarters of the city. It is so uncomplicated to stop by for a cup of tea with these families and exchange a few words. They treasure these encounters, and a friendly relationship with a few of them has developed over time. Therefore, Christian Schneider's understanding of humanity and God appeals to me. But he'll hardly appear at my door because of this.

I'll fly back to the Philippines again the day after tomorrow. The saying about laughing and weeping eyes is hackneyed, but it fits. Consequently, I'm happy all the more that a bit of Switzerland will accompany me to Manila: The medical nurse, Regula Hauser, and the epidemiologist, Christian Auer, will travel with me to live in the slums, and later presumably Regina and Markus Meyer and their three children will follow. Quite courageous! We are now the official "envoys" of the newly founded Servants Switzerland.

We plan to publish a newsletter now and then. We owe it to our friends and patrons to report on developments, successes, and failures.

I've been waiting for two months perhaps to hear from Christian, and now he actually does call me, two days before he is to return to Manila, and asks if I would be willing to publish a newsletter every few months to be sent to contributors. Admittedly, a somewhat more romantic question would also have been welcome... but still! Given the circumstances, what more can I expect other than regular mail from Christian from Manila?

Christine actually agreed spontaneously and without much deliberation. She sounded really enthused. Did her agreement suggest more of an interest in the work of Servants or in me? Well, fine, whatever. She is a fascinating person and will certainly be a very good colleague. At least that . . .

The Corpses Will Be Buried Later

October 1990. Approaching land at the Manila International Airport. I've been on my feet for over twenty-four hours already but am nevertheless still wide awake. My head is full of thoughts. A half year in Switzerland lies behind me with many incredible encounters with great people. In front of me lies my second home, the slums, with incredibly many encounters with great people. I can now connect Basel with Bagong Silang and Potrero, and from now on the Servants in Switzerland, as an organization, will support and shape this connection.

I am immensely happy that in a short time, even in Manila, I will hear the trusty Swiss dialect. In the beginning, Regula and Christian will live in the Servants team house. Later they will also move to domicile in a slum. I've known Regula a long time; we worked together in the University Hospital in Basel. In 1988 she spent two months with the poor in Manila and determined to settle there one day. Christian finished writing his thesis for his diploma from the Tropical Institute a long time ago, but after his visit to me two years ago, he couldn't get the slums out of his mind. Now he wants to combine his work as a slum worker with his doctoral dissertation about health in the slums. Splendid!

I am heartily welcomed in Potrero and Bagong Silang. I visit my little "worlds" and bring myself up-to-date on how things stand, including information about the earthquake. It happened two and a half months ago, and 1,621 people were killed. Thankfully, none of my friends or acquaintances were affected.

Many are still involved and active in our "Orphanage," that began with the bodyguards, and which we renovated at the end of the last year. Others couldn't withstand the bad influence of friends and need our intervention, especially Reymond and Mata with his new name, Brian. The chicken cultivation project is more bad than good. In contrast, the activities of the youth group are running well, as are the communal living arrangements that have developed. Of course, there is too much turnover of pastors, and actually there are none at the moment. Albert's alphabet class was over at the end of the school year; Brian, Datu, and Jessy can read and write. The clinic, overseen by Dr. Jo, a physician from New Zealand, is more than over burdened.

A few days after my return, a friend from the Diliman Bible Church (DBC), a Filipino middle-class church, arrives. A Christian community in the earthquake area asked his church for help, and they were now organizing a quick-response effort. The region surrounding the epicenter, which is desperately poor and miserably inaccessible, is correspondingly neglected by the government—even in earthquake assistance. I offer my services and can provide a number of men from our slum areas to work with us. Help is necessary: The better the living situation in the provinces, the smaller the possibility of new refugees in the slums of the capital.

Now I am lying flat on the roof of a truck, enjoying the wind of the road, and the good feeling of traveling together. I'm most happy that both the indigenous rich and the poor are working together. I am the only Caucasian in this delegation of approximately twenty helpers. After a few hours we begin to slow down. We're approaching the mountainous region. Bridges and segments of roads are destroyed; we frequently have to drive around them, with difficulty. Our goal of the day is to cross the Dalton Pass on the north-south supply axis of the main island of Luzon. The earthquake loosed landslides and earth displacements and the axis was closed for weeks. Grain, vegetables, and fruits from the hinterland were able to reach the markets in Manila only by detour, which drove the prices up.

Night has fallen as we finally reach our lodgings, a beautifully appointed mission station of the "New Tribes Mission," in the middle of a vast hilly landscape. A good 10,000 people live here, spread among widely dispersed settlements. The quaking as well as torrential rain destroyed entire rice fields, coffee and cacao plantations, and other plantings. "It will be two or three years before the farmers in these mountains will be able to take care of themselves again," says a man at the mission station who is working with us.

The next morning we begin before the sun rises. Local porters from the surrounding villages load the mules and themselves with giant packages of supplies on their brown shoulders and strong heads. A young lady from the DBC requisitions a mule to ride. This angers me, but I don't have the nerve to criticize her.

I notice another young lady in our delegation from a quite different perspective. First of all, she is very bright and second, markedly beautiful . . . the latter of which I notice first, logically, since one sees with one's eyes after all. Her name is Dorie Morden, a Filipina, who is in charge of logistics on this endeavor. She is well-educated and practically gifted. And I'm particularly pleased that the church that she attends is not far from our Servants team house.

The march is not a pleasure. We plod and slide many long hours over roads and sludge channels. The weeks-long monsoon made them completely sodden. Except for a couple of shrubs and coconut palms, the landscape is almost completely barren. Earlier the volcanic earth of this region was held together by the strong roots of the rain forests, I am told. Then, with complete disregard, the Spanish conquerors and later the industrialists deforested the area. Since then dangerous landslides are not unusual in the rain season.

We take a longer break beside a stream, put our feet up, and fill plastic bags with drinking water. I have chlorine tablets that I now dissolve in the water; up here in this secluded area, diarrhea is the last thing that I need. My aching shoulders are enough already. "We'll be there presently," the guides say again and again. In the meantime, however, I have enough experience to know what "presently" means: namely anything between five minutes and five hours.

Filthy and tired as dogs, we arrive in a larger village shortly before nightfall. Laughing children take us to a kind of schoolhouse made from bamboo and corrugated tin. After a shower, consisting of a plastic bucket full of water with a tin can, and a meal of fresh rice and chicken, I feel better again. The people are incredibly hospitable.

Our leaders discuss with the village elders how best the supplies should be distributed. Some sick people show up, from somewhere. We have a Filipino doctor with our group whom I help care for the patients in the light of a gasoline lamp. There are cases of diarrhea, bronchitis, and some wounds to be treated. Nonetheless, the people here seem much fresher and healthier than my neighbors in the slums of the large metropolis.

Later in the night, over a hundred people gather for a thanksgiving service. Their gratitude moves me. Evidently we are the first to bring help, except for a visit by a government helicopter, which left behind some groceries, a few medications, and many empty promises. The people sing about Jesus, and their faces glow with joy. Their faith overwhelms me; it is so straightforward and sincere. The happiness caused by our arrival is naturally also a reason for their spontaneous thanksgiving service. Nevertheless one senses that the people really find consolation in their faith.

The distribution of the goods is a major event. The gratitude of the residents of these remote villages without streets, electricity, or telephone allows one to quickly forget the exertion involved. We distribute to approximately 1,800 families eleven tons of rice, three tons of milk powder, three tons of sugar, seven sacks of salt, mungo beans, 2,000 tins of sardines, and 1,200 pieces of clothing. More than 400 patients receive medications. For future use, we distribute several hundred pounds of seed (rice and vegetables), tools, and 400 pounds of nails.

In one settlement of 170 families, the quake had destroyed the irrigation system of all four of their rice fields. We buy the material for its replacement.

In another settlement, the quake changed the course of a river so that the water supply to life-sustaining fish ponds for the population dried up. We encourage them to re-channel the river's course and give them the necessary packets of nourishment for each workday. We contribute 15,000 franks toward the total from the Swiss Aid Account.

The way home is more pleasant, shoulders and hearts are lighter. Finally we arrive in an unobstructed area. With two others, I can ride in an open Jeep. We have a bumpy ride ahead of us, but after a long march on foot, climbing into a motor vehicle again is a small deliverance. Five hours later, it is pitch black.

Our driver, Freddy, has a tried and true antidote to fatigue: driving faster. Suddenly we see in the cone of the headlights, for a fraction of a second, two human bodies lying on the side of the road. And, I believe that they were covered in blood.

"They are wounded; stop, Freddy!" I shout.

"No, they are dead; and it's none of our business!"

"But we should maybe help," I add, intimidated.

"Much too dangerous," Freddy answers, and keeps his foot on the gas pedal.

A few silent minutes later we see several people standing at an intersection. Freddy stops, and dismayed, we tell them about our discovery. "Yes, yes, but they are dead," one says, as if this were the most usual thing in the world. "Two motorcycle riders who were felled by a truck. The corpses will be buried later."

On the trip remaining, I say not a word. I long for the familiarity of our slum home.

Paulo

With every word and deed, I became aware how absurd it seems for a Swiss to feel at home in a slum as I noticed how people in Switzerland reacted to me. One is instantly perceived as a bit ludicrous, a bit of an example, a bit of a hero. At the same time, the slum is not my home; rather it has to do with my relationship to the people therein. It's about discovering who they are without allowing the loathsome aspects of the slums to drive one away. The stable in Bethlehem stank too.

Regula and Christian appear to adjust well in their new slums. Christian lives with a family in Frisco, Regula is with a family of eight in Batasan. She has abruptly changed her name to Rachel, for in the Philippines Regula means menstruation. . . . We Swiss meet once a week in the Servants team house, together with Elizabeth, a Swiss national who works for another missionary community. Beyond that we see each other every three weeks at the so-called Team time which, for the time being, lasts from Wednesday afternoon until Friday morning. Some twenty-five Servants in all participate in Team time, thirteen of them children.

Today I met with Dorie Morden. There is more than simply empathy on both sides. She is the same age as I am, studied at the University of the Philippines and received a Master's degree. She is currently the headmistress of a number of kindergartens. That's how she supports herself. One can tell that she's of the upper middle class. We are in love now, it's obvious—but where to go from here? I'm a little out of character, playing this role. Which role, actually? What *is* my role?

I am a missionary, development aide, and idealist. Naturally, rumors circulate here and there about the foreigner who chats with the children in the alleys and plays with them. Some have a suspicion that I'm one of the white pedophiles about which warnings are broadcast on television. Others think that I'm a CIA agent who is hiding in the slums. Even here the people watch too much TV.

In any case, Ate Donita has assured me that she trusts me again. My hardheaded reluctance to come to her Bible study class made her uncertain. But the next morning she prayed that God would tell her the truth about me, "and then I dusted your little room. A cat jumped down from the cupboard and knocked a cardboard box to the floor. As I put the papers back in the box, I saw your diploma from a Bible College in England and your ordination certificate when you were made pastor. Then I was relieved."

Late at night I lie in my quarters and ponder what I should write for the new Servants newspaper. It should be good since Christine will oversee it, and she is a teacher. But I won't be the only one who will write reports. Christian and Regula will also have an abundance of stories to tell. Good. I always have too little time for everything, anyway.

With one ear I overhear the goings on in the life of Jeffry and Rosalie. They both live with their children Albin and Mona directly behind one of my four plywood walls. Jeffry is one of Ate Donita's difficult, fatherless sons. The young couple work nights in a nightclub, as dancers and who knows what else. They usually sleep during the day.

Ate Donita asked me already some time ago to talk with her son. "They don't listen to me anymore. Their lifestyle is going to kill them one of these days." Originally, Jeffry studied optometry, and both of them had even made a start in trusting Jesus. But, Ate Donita told me, one year before the end of his studies, everything came apart. The money ran out, Rosalie became pregnant, and the reaction of the church congregation was everything but helpful. It was then that they began their degrading work at the nightclub, which they've already been doing for two years.

As I think about Rosalie and Jeffry, Ate Donita suddenly bursts into the room: "Chris, my brother is spitting blood and is possessed by demons!" Fear is written on her face.

She goes ahead of me, and I follow her. I know her brother Paulo only casually, and I don't really like him. He is one of those diseased fathers who don't care for their families and instead with an insolent grin, agitate and provoke, are unapproachable, unappealing, and unreliable, always searching for material, clients, or customers. A few huts further, we climb up a dirty ladder and into a tiny apartment. Paulo lies on a thin mat, his breathing is short and heaving, and he glows with sweat and shivers at the same time. His wife, Miriam, and his flock of children stare at me.

"Do something!" Ate Donita implores. "He went to see a quack who hit him in the stomach with a strange cane and infused him with a black liquid. Now he's coughing up blood and hair and other gruesome things."

The belief in spirits is present everywhere; to speak of spirits here does not seem odd, the way it does in Europe. Therefore I explain to Paulo that Jesus Christ is much stronger than all spirits and powers. Then we say a short prayer for the exorcising of all evil spirits and for the healing of his apparent tuberculosis that has broken through. I can't do more at the moment. As we depart, Paulo seems somewhat calmer.

The next day Paulo steps into my partition, sits down and begins to speak. I don't understand everything but that doesn't matter. He is ridding himself of a kind of life confession. For ten years, he has followed many crooked roads and criminal paths in order to acquire his drug, crystal meth, and to this end has offered up the well-being of his wife, Miriam, and his four children. I tell him about God, who loves all humanity and gladly forgives them so that they can achieve peace. Paulo wants to accept this forgiveness. We pray again.

In the evening on my mat, I let this moment pass by again for review and savor it. No one can take the experience of the power of prayer away from me. Prayer is overwhelming. And in the meantime, Paulo seems more likeable to me.

A week later Paulo and I meet for the third time for conversation with black coffee and sweets. This time he brings four friends along. They all want to give up drugs. Paulo appears to have inspired them. We read the Bible, pray, discuss. There's also much to laugh about—my stumbling Tagalog is still highly entertaining. But above all, it is exciting how the lights go on for these men and they suddenly produce confessions and can admit the truth about themselves. One can sense how liberating communal prayer is for them.

"The Bible says that Christians should have fellowship with each other," I tell the men. They nod. We determine to search for an appropriate church in Potrero. I don't want to join Ate Donita's Ladies Circle, however. Definitely not. This little awakening with the men is super, but I won't allow myself to be taken over to the degree that I was in Bagong Silang.

Today Dorie and I took a walk on the campus of her university. She is quite proud of her Master's degree. Last week we visited her uncle, a rich fisherman. His considerable fishing grounds are "fenced in" with nets. Armed guards stand ready with guns loaded in order to shoot the poor who would dare to approach the nets with knives to steal fish. Dorie is proud of her rich relations. But perhaps it's only a demonstration for me, since I myself belong to the "rich,"—or, to smother the underlying suspicion that she is interested in me above all because of my "riches." Whatever. In any case, she is quite in love. And I'm somewhat confused.

I have to admit to myself that I sometimes feel very lonely. One would think quite the contrary in a world in which one is constantly surrounded by people. I can bear the lack of roast potatoes, and I have the opportunity to speak my own language now and then. It's not just the color of my skin, but rather much more importantly, the foreign culture. It's the life left behind with all the relationships in a world that simply doesn't exist for my friends here. I have experienced some moments of inner strife in the last three years.

Unfulfilled sexuality plays a part: the attempt to live as a bachelor in a warm climate and in an area in which sex is one of the few regular free entertainments available. For this reason, I don't experience the enormous sensuality of the Philippine culture as helpful.

At least another peculiarity of the South Asian culture comes to my aid in being single, namely the emotionally charged friendships between men. They grow spontaneously, wherever one travels together or works together. In the beginning I had to become accustomed to an unfamiliar physical proximity. Filipinos have no inhibitions about touching each other everywhere at every opportunity. Also among men the spontaneous expression of feelings is not only allowed but normal. In the meantime, not only have I grown accustomed to it, but have discovered how enriching this kind of relationship is in the world of men.

Of course, the question of fulfilled sexuality remains unanswered. In any case, the longer it continues the less sure I am if I want to or am able to lead my celibate life for an extended period of time.

Rico, the Resolute

March 1991, four months have passed. What's happening here in Potrero is fabulous! When I ask Paulo how he's doing at work, he proudly shows me the callouses on his hands. In December, as his new beginning seemed to me to be ongoing, I gave him a small loan with which he then repaired an old motorbike with a sidecar. And now, not quite five months since that memorable evening when he lay half dead on his mat, he earns his money honestly with his motorbike taxi and also brings it home, rather than to a drug dealer. Paulo's joy in life is flowing from every pore.

A regular dialogue-and-prayer-circle has grown out of our sporadic meetings. The last time I had fifteen men in my partition—that is, crowded in front of my open door; fellows with tattoos, scars, and other traces of life, with bad manners and meager vocabulary, but above all with the will for a new beginning without drugs.

Yesterday I sent a particularly impressive story to Christine Tanner for our little Swiss Servants newspaper, namely about Boboy, the worst of all "my" men. Boboy has killed four people and has spent a substantial part of his life in the ugly prisons of Manila. In Potrero he is considered "the godfather" of drug addicts. When the thirty-two-year-old appeared here a few weeks ago, he looked like a skeleton. He suffered from tuberculosis and needed a "hit" three times a day. I told him that if he allowed Jesus into his life, everything would be changed. I hope he didn't notice that I had doubts myself if he could be helped.

In any case, Boboy is still alive; he lives night and day in a 3 ft. x 6 ft. "rehab room." We organized an around-the-clock watch. Thereby the risk that he leaves to get drugs is diminished. He survived the withdrawal. As before, his state of health is critical, but I am more optimistic than before.

Fortunately everything is not my responsibility. I got Pepe Gonzales involved, the youth pastor with whom I organized a few good youth camps and who also came along to Snake Island. Pepe is a former engineer who was re-educated as a pastor, and is an engaged, enthusiastic person. His mother owns a small fish-sauce factory, and Pepe has few financial worries. He lives with his family an hour toward the north, in Navotas. This suburb of Manila has about double as many residents as Basel, but is only about one third as large. Pepe often stops by in Potrero. When our new friends have special concerns or need prayers, I sometimes refer them to Pepe.

From the beginning, Ate Donita has also played a key role. She oversees and controls self-help projects. Thereby I more or less protect myself from myself, because Ate Donita's oversight prevents me from handing over money to help someone. Cash creates dependencies; one's interventions must be administered in proper doses. Whenever I see a way, I try to avoid this through a go-between.

The question of money is a great challenge because the men need new sources of income when they give up thievery, mugging, and drug dealing. Without intending to, I have now and again furthered self-help projects. In the meantime we have established numerous bicycle and motorbike taxis, a chicken farm, and a small sheet-metal workshop.

In addition, we want to build a small chapel, not as a signal of taking over a district as established religions did or still do, but rather for pragmatic reasons. I had planned to integrate "my" men in local churches since a Christian should seek to be in fellowship. Consequently we attended services in various churches. The result was disillusioning: The well-behaved faithful eyed the men anxiously or surveyed them with pity as they entered the churches with their tattoos and scars and their, shall we say, *unconvential* manners. Then they sat down and were lectured by preachers who liked to hear themselves talk and whose monologues clearly implied that if one lived as a Christian, one did well, and those who remained poor were doing something wrong. In other words, not exactly what we read together in the Bible about the poor, Jesus, and his followers.

So we didn't have much choice other than to become a small church ourselves. Romeo, one of our former gangsters, has a piece of land on which the chapel is to be built. I'm looking forward to it in joyful anticipation. It will be a chapel in which men who bear tattoos rather than manners are expressly welcome.

Today I was in Bagong Silang again, and visited my boys, Brian and Reymond, and the others. There are, to be sure, setbacks, but in sum, my projects in my very first slum bring me joy. Albert's class has also grown, and his students advance.

As I return and climb off my Honda, a stranger stands before me, a man about thirty. He immediately gets to the point: His name is Rico and he wants to turn his back on everything that is evil. For years he was a member of a drug syndicate in Bagong Barrio and took part in robberies and muggings. Although he's pretty well off financially, he leads a failed life and is constantly afraid. His old gang members want to kill him because he is no longer a part of the gang. He has a lot of enemies and it has become too dangerous for him in Bagong Barrio. Finally, he also has a family, a son from his first marriage and now also a child with his second wife.

I am unsure about what I think of him. The man is slightly built, but he makes a good impression; he speaks fluently and lucidly. Resolutely, he comes to the point: He had earlier made sandals and sold them; he is a good craftsman and would like to begin with this honest work. He has heard that we would make loans available. He would also read the Bible and pray if this were required of him.

Rico's unusually purposeful behavior makes an impression on me. On the other hand, his appearance has something macho about it. He lives in a small slum settlement on a former cemetery plot in another part of the city. Here in my own slum, life is more or less transparent; here I know the people or I know people who know the people—but I can't judge whether Rico's story is true.

"We must first get to know each other," I finally say. "You certainly understand that I cannot simply trust every stranger. In reference to a loan, I can only make a recommendation. The decision lies with Ate Donita and our Church committee."

The next day I ask several of my friends who "earn" their money in Potrero as drug dealers if they know Rico. They nod vigorously: He is a dangerous man from a dangerous gang; whatever happens, I must be careful. Help! What should I do?

Faith for Cash

Dorie and I "called it quits," as one says so nicely, actually before we really began a relationship. The cultural differences are simply too great. We decided this during a stroll together. Dorie was visibly disappointed, but I am sure that it's good as it is. Beginning a relationship with a Servants' worker would not be easy; a complete identification with the Servants philosophy has to be present in order for it to work. Living in the slums is not for everyone.

Last evening I was out late again. That usually happens when I visit Bagong Silang. The boys from the "Orphanage" keep one trotting. Our walk-in clinic is also still open, as before. Jo, a physician from New Zealand, runs it. But she wants to stop and become more involved in health education for children instead. Regula Hauser is pondering whether she should take over the assignment.

In any case, I spent the night in Bagong Silang. As I returned to Potrero in the morning, the first thing that I discover is a spray of blood on the plywood door of my lodgings. Ate Donita is already there. "Fortunately you were away! A bomb exploded in front of your door! Two of us are in the hospital, severely wounded. Fortunately Lola Lucia got hit lightly, in the legs."

An attack on my lodgings? I swallow. That gives me pause. It was a nail bomb, clearly homemade, like those used in gang wars. It is consisted of explosives, nails, and metal fragments. One throws it like a hand grenade at one's opponent. As it strikes the ground, the nails and metal fragments inside hit one another and produce tiny sparks that are enough to cause the explosives to detonate.

"Does anybody know who threw the bomb?" I ask Ate Donita.

"Nobody," she says, and reports what happened. Jeffry and Rosalie had decided to move to another part of the city, away from the drug scene in Potrero, from life as "dancers," and from their families with their constant complaints. During the move, two friends carried their clothes cupboard down the wobbly stairs. The cupboard tilted to the side, the slum house construction began to totter, and a nail bomb rolled off the wooden beam above my small roof to the floor, and exploded.

It wasn't an attack, but nonetheless. Someone hid a bomb in my space, most probably because the risk of finding it here was minimal—a police raid on my place is inconceivable. Well thought out. Nevertheless it's hair brained to hide a bomb that explodes upon impact six feet above the floor. Who could that have been? Maybe I've been living with a bomb in my room for months? But then it explodes during my absence. I shudder.

Now two severely wounded people lie in the hospital, and Jeffry and Rosalie will have to come up with the money for the hospital bill. They'll have to earn money again as quickly as possible. In the nightclub—where else? Their cupboard stands, even though damaged, in its former place. The end of their new beginning. Oh, God!

In the afternoon I visit Rico in his cemetery domicile. Only when I have met his wife and children will I be able to judge if I can trust him. I come upon a wretched, but clean living space in the middle of graves—a kind of hide out. Both of them welcome me warmly. Rico's wife tells me about the life of their family and begins to weep. She verifies Rico's story as credible. Apparently he really does want to begin anew. Rico shows me a pair of sandals that he made and again tells me of his plans.

On the one hand, I trust Rico. On the other hand, the thought that in concept we are beginning to be perceived as something like a lending institution disturbs me—that any kind of strange people can turn up, particularly because of the money. I am undecided. But suddenly I have an idea.

"Rico," I say, "you were a drug dealer and gangster and now want to become a trusted merchant. First you have to prove to me that you're serious about the faith. If you're able to do that, to come to services every Sunday for three months, I will thereafter recommend you to our committee for a loan."

Rico laughs. "Not only I, but my whole family will now be there in Potrero."

On the way home it suddenly becomes clear to me what kind of bargain I had just made: Money for faith. I am an idiot! I've been living here for almost three years and have actually learned that such linkages bring nothing other than people who become "Christians" for economic reasons. And now I wade into this waterfall like someone who has not the slightest idea about mission and development assistance. Or like one of those preachers who believe that as a Christian one does well, and poverty is a sign that one is doing something wrong. I feel a little sick.

Four days after the bomb explosion Jeffry approaches me and speaks to me more openly than ever before. In despair he tells me that he has been searching for Rosalie for two whole days and that she was being held captive by a narcotics ring. She was being set up by the men dealing in cocaine, naturally under pressure and under the strong influence of drugs. "A syndicate boss held a pistol to my head and warned me not to get involved in the Rosalie situation." They had pretended to be sister and brother at the nightclub.

I have no idea what to do and simply listen to him. Then I ask him if I should pray for him and Rosalie. He nods and we pray together. When one doesn't know what to do, praying is best. Above all, here one isn't immediately looked at askance as in Western Europe, where most people only pray in phrases, if at all, with the children at the table or before going to sleep, and where calling someone "devout" is an insult. I find the matter-of-course, comfortable attitude toward praying here in the slums very liberating.

The next day Rosalie turns up. She has lost all of her strength. "Go to Navotas to Pastor Pepe," I say. And they do, together with Rosalie's mother.

On the same evening, a message reaches me that my father has died.

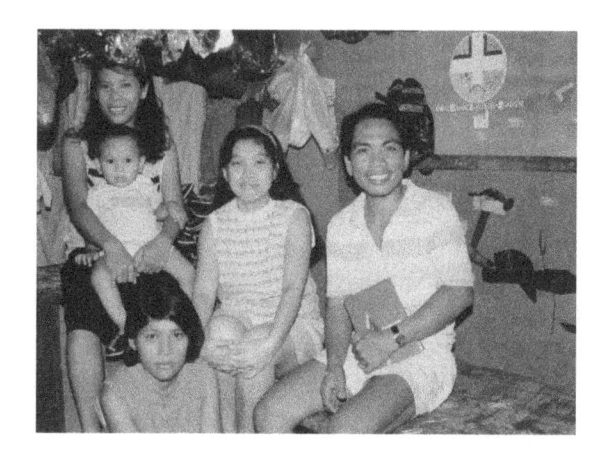

The former gangster Rico with his family in his hiding place in a graveyard; in his hand, a Bible, and on his face, a new smile.

Navotas

It is a confusion of feelings. The arrival in Switzerland, overcome, torn away from my world. The moments at the coffin. My siblings, my mother, the funeral, which have unexpectedly set me back into my childhood. And I'm already sitting in an airplane again, watching absentmindedly as the stewardesses demonstrate the use of a life vest and oxygen mask. A cocktail of feelings.

Sometimes in the evening when we were in bed, my father would play something for us on his harmonica. He also liked to sing. He seldom spoke of his work as a nurse in a psychiatric clinic, and when he did, it was about his dissatisfaction. If he was taking his midday nap or listening to the news on the radio, we all had to be quiet. He has a difficult job, our weary mother would often offer as an excuse. Particularly she, who gave birth in less than six years to as many children and who without household help mastered an immense task. In hindsight it becomes clear: I really didn't know him.

He had a unique story. His father grew up as a child laborer in the impoverished Swiss area of Emmenthal, and at the turn of the century had to seek his survival as a farmhand in foreign Germany. He settled near the Baltic Sea, where my father then also grew up, together with seventeen siblings and half-siblings. Like everyone else, he belonged to the Hitler Youth, and toward the end of the Second World War joined the navy as a volunteer, practically still a child. At the age of seventeen, thanks to a Swiss passport, he could emigrate to Switzerland. One can only imagine: A Northern German Hitler youth and "child soldier," seventeen-years-old, in Switzerland. Presumably, my father felt like a homeless person during his life.

The humid Philippine heat in Manila tears me away from my trip to the past back to the present. Also in Bagong Silang and Potrero, children have to put themselves out to service, the member codes of the gangs are so strict and totalitarian as those of the Hitler Youth, homelessness and life's struggles are everyday events, many "emigrate" to drugs: alcohol, glue sniffing, or crystal meth. There is much to do.

The next day, after more than an hour of difficult driving through the glowing city, I get off my Honda in front of Pepe's family home. Already several times, Pepe asked me to become a presence with the Servants in the slums of his suburb Navotas. Navotas lies on the Bay of Manila and is completely overcrowded. Twice previously we have provided a one-day medical clinic in one of the slums. Now I want to speak and pray with Pepe about the possible work of the Servants in Navotas.

I knock. A maid opens the door. "The Gonzales family has gone to the Provinces for a few days," she says. Drat! That means three hours of city traffic for nothing.

I thank her. But rather than climbing back onto the Honda, I take off on foot, since if I'm already here, I can simply visit the people of the neighboring slum. The slum lies between a rubbish dump and a cemetery. Many hundreds of families live there in cramped space. On the ocean side they have built their shacks on bamboo stilts out over the water; on land the settlement grows directly into the colony of graves. The mausoleums with their walled-in corpses serve as supporting walls for the homes of some of the residents. What I see here, however, hits me like a hammer: One of the hurricanes during recent days has damaged the slum massively. Many shacks on bamboo stilts have been torn apart by the wind, or transported into the ocean in one piece. The area is covered with a dirty blanket of slime. Using cloth, cardboard, and plastic planks the people try to shield themselves from rain. The stench is deplorable. Bones and skulls lie about—the storm has apparently opened a number of graves, perhaps the improvised graves of the poor. Helplessness and sadness come over me.

Naked, dirty, and undernourished children run toward me and touch me. The approach to the shacks lies six to ten feet over the slimy beach and consists of destroyed, slippery bamboo stalks. A dangerous home, not only for the children. I speak to a few people. They are not only tired and despondent, but also feel abandoned by the rest of the world and especially by their government.

A family remembers me from one of my day clinics and presses me to enter their improvised rice-sack construction. They bring me a cool cola and a few cookies from somewhere. Heavens! I try to refrain but without success. I cannot and may not refuse; it would be the rudest incivility to decline these gestures of hospitality. I have to drink, and every sip is torture when I think about the fact that the money for the cola most likely was to have been sufficient for supper for the family. The mother says that she belongs to the fourteen families whose entire huts, including contents, were lost in the floods. One child drowned.

On the way home, my feelings alternate among rage, shock, and violent emotion. I have to speak to Pepe, to see what we can do. In the following days I organize some photos and send them together with a report to my friends in Switzerland. Why, ultimately, did we found Servants Switzerland anyway?

At the moment I do not worry about the distribution of aid. Pepe began to form a network of relationships years ago. A couple of capable women meet regularly to barter and to read the Bible. He knows them and can trust them. I think of Ate Donita and her circle of women. Women pray more than men. Men drink more than women and are more often drug addicted. Apparently it is easier for women to admit neediness, to ask for help and to accept it, while men in need founder. That's why I don't like the arrogant demeanor of many men.

In the evening I read a letter from my friend Peter, a young doctor from Switzerland. He asks me about my observations regarding issues of over population. I will tell him that in my view, so-called over population is not the main reason for, but rather a result of, poverty.

Of course, I experience daily how families are overwhelmed in almost every respect by their many children. The resulting tragedies that arise create the intrinsic drama in the life and death of the poor. But after three years in the slum I know that the people here don't comprehend how I can speak about something such as "family planning" as long as their children die of harmless children's sicknesses and diarrhea. They naturally see it from another perspective: The more children they have, the greater the chance that some will survive.

Besides, family planning requires protection measures, that is, the money for them. And discipline; and the nerve to resist the teachings of the Catholic Church, which notably rejects artificial protection as an act against God's dominion over life and death. (Whereby, according to this logic they would also have to be against medical help).

My poor neighbors have enough to do just to survive. Leisure activities or self-development are simply not in the picture. In the slum the essential things for which life is worth living are religion, food, sex, and togetherness with one's own family. To identify the great number of children of the poor as a basis for poverty is far too simple. Above all, although people in the First World point their fingers at the over-sized families of the poor, it's really their lifestyle that burdens natural resources a hundred times more than the lifestyle of people in the Third World. Again, a reason to lie awake at night.

Two Angels and a Motorcycle

Boboy is gone. He probably fell back into his old life. I am angry, hurt, sad. That simply cannot be! So many people who took such an interest in him, protected him, prayed with him, took care of him. Should we search for him, or should we leave it at praying for him?

This afternoon I do something that I've wanted to do for a long time: I force myself to go to a closed off part of Potrero about which Ate Donita and Lola Lucia warned me in unison, saying that it is inhabited by the most violent alcoholics of the worst kind imaginable.

Walking around, I see a normal slum quarter of forty to fifty shacks—many children, women washing clothes, a few old people and naturally, as usual, also a couple of men who are drinking. Quite a few know me already and seem amused that I am for once also looking in on their corner. Someone leads me to a simple wooden shack built on stilts. We go in.

A sick man is lying on a cloth on the floor. I sit down next to him. As my eyes adjust to the half-darkness and I look closely, I am frightened. The man is in pitiful shape, looking as if he is dying. I'm not prepared for this. He has yellow eyes, is thin as a skeleton and short of breath. Tuberculosis. With the greatest of difficulty, he succeeds in sitting up. It's impossible to gauge his age.

He can barely speak, but is happy about my visit. Jojie is his name, he says. He has no one except for his old mother, since people were naturally afraid that he would infect them. However, he did receive food from the neighbors again and again; otherwise, he and his mother would have starved. I know that almost all of the residents in this slum quarter come from the same province in the southern Philippines. Their solidarity is therefore more pronounced than elsewhere. He has heard of us, Jojie whispers, and when he gets better and he can walk again, he would attend our fellowship meeting.

I sit here, at the limit of my possibilities, at the side of a deathly ill man my age who speaks of a time when he will be better. I doubt that in his condition time in a clinic would make any difference. Helpless, I ask again if I should pray with him. He nods. We pray.

Some days later I am riding my Honda in the direction of Bagong Silang. As often before, I approach through Tala, the leper colony. About halfway there something peculiar crosses my field of vision, and I stop. On the horizon in an otherwise blue sky, a mighty cloud rises up. In the bright midday sun it glows like a giant silver-gray cauliflower. Incredibly beautiful, but also threatening. A very atypical thundercloud of the nimbus variety. I mount my bike and rumble further along the unpaved road. I have to quickly accomplish only the most pressing tasks in Bagong Silang and head back, before the tropical thunder breaks through!

Shortly thereafter I stop a second time because my back wheel is swerving. I discover that I have a flat tire. Ah, splendid! In the city of Manila there is a tire repair shop on every corner, but out here, just before Tala. . . . I have a substitute tube with me, also a multi-purpose wrench and screwdriver, but it's not enough for a back tire-tube change including sprocket-wheel mounting, brake drum, and gears. I am a fool. Brooding midday heat, anticipated thunder, a 270-pound motorcycle to push, and not a single person on the street! I've been on my way not even five minutes, panting and sweating, when two figures appear. They laugh—not at me, of that I'm sure. In this culture people react to almost everything with an audible laugh, even when the situation isn't funny. Perhaps it's a kind of emotional release?

"Don't worry," one of them says, "we'll mend your bike, just wait a little while." The other one scurries away, presumably to get help. Will this go well? Both their faces are disfigured by leprosy. A few minutes later the second man is back, with various screwdrivers, pliers, and an air pump. Now both strange angels begin to work. . . . I am dreadfully embarrassed. They won't allow me to help, but I can't convince them to stop. I notice that leprosy has also maimed their fingers. They've gotten the wheel out of the frame, are removing brake and gear shafts, and try with much effort to loosen the hub from the wheel rim. They lose their grip again and again and injure themselves on the sharp metal edges—one can't stand by and watch any longer! Their truncated fingers begin to bleed, and I would love to sink into the earth. Both employ hands and feet, and suffer sprains as they work, but refuse to let me help. Each second seems like an eternity to me.

It's incredible, but the men manage to fix my motorcycle. They get up and look at me beaming, happy and proud of their victory over the machine, over the situation, perhaps also over the ravages of their illness. They, the poor sick men at the edge of the road, and I, the healthy white man—with a motorcycle that must be worth a fortune in their eyes. Once again this inversion of the world with its values. These two have shattered every cliché, exactly as the one born in a stable shattered clichés.

Of course they now also refuse to allow me to thank them. This time, however, I am stubborn even though I only have some small change with me. If I had a fortune with me, I would have left it for them—they gave me everything that they had. Finally they do accept the small change and laugh. Grateful but upset, I drive on.

By 3:00 o'clock in the afternoon I'm back in the city. It's getting darker and darker. Irritated, I look at my watch again, but I'm not mistaken; it really is only 3:00 o'clock in the afternoon. Now the streetlights are actually coming on. Strange. As I climb off the motor bike with a stiff back at home in Potrero, it begins to snow. Now a light goes on in my head, and the first person that I meet confirms my thought: This morning Pinatubo erupted. Because of an "atypical thunder cloud of the nimbus variety," meteorologist Schneider mistook a volcanic eruption for thunder.

In a very short time everything is covered with a layer of white ash. The Pinatubo is located barely sixty miles from us. The cloud of ash was fourteen miles high, they are saying on television, and within just a few hours had swallowed the sunlight of the greater part of the island.

Powerful. In the evening, on my plank-bed, I have an empty feeling in the pit of my stomach. End-time, somehow. A rain of ashes, the darkening day, and then the appearance of two leper angels. I will never forget the theological lesson of these two as long as I live: It is not easy to accept help from someone who seems helpless. Neither from lepers nor from the one born in a stable.

Tired

Together with about fifty other women and men I am sitting at a religious service, and I am happy. About three weeks ago, we dedicated our new chapel and already it seems too small. A good sign. But I am happy for other reasons—for example, because Rico is sitting with the congregation. He no longer commits robberies; instead he is a small businessman with a sandal workshop, built with the loan that Ate Donita's committee gave him. Now as before, he comes to the service with his family, and I have noticed that he also reads his large Bible at home, and so consistently that I have seldom seen its like in my experience.

I am also happy that Boboy is here again. He came back. And I'm happy about Rosalie and Jeffry and their two small children. Rosalie stands in the front and tells how she formerly sold herself to the nightclub and to cocaine and at the end actually consumed crystal meth, but some time ago began a new life with the help of Jesus Christ. Wow!

Yesterday Pepe was able to baptize thirty people in a river outside the city. Among them was the elderly Papa Dela Cruz, Jeffry's grandfather, the authority figure of Potrero. Everything was very smooth and impressive—unheard of, I was told. I stayed away from the Baptism on purpose. In this predominantly Catholic land, I don't particularly want to be known as the Baptist. It was a simple opportunity to demonstrate that everything functions very well without me. The longer I am here, the more important this is to me.

Ate Donita told me recently that long before my first visit in Potrero, her Ladies Circle had the impression while praying that an Amerikano would come to show their men the way to faith and to help them out of their addiction. She logically connected that with me. Clearly, I feel flattered; who doesn't like to feel as if he's "called upon." Otherwise, the role of the Messiah doesn't suit me, which was also my reason for staying away from the Baptism. If I were seen as "the bringer of blessings," what I represent and want would be betrayed. But Ate Donita is completely convinced, and I let the matter rest. Nonetheless, I am grateful to this conviction which prompted her to offer the Amerikano who arrived on the scene one day lodging and hospitality so readily.

"My" men are happy to come to the services in our new chapel; our regular meetings are more absorbing and intensive than before. It has little to do with me, however; rather, it's because of the long and faithful prayers of the women that prepared the groundwork. I am convinced of that.

In the evening I lie pondering on my plank bed. How will it continue with these faithful? I don't know. Most of them are lacking in every way: employment possibilities; medical care; money for children's schooling; inhuman living situations; etc. Again, much care and patience is necessary, so that we don't arrive too quickly with immediate help and awaken the impression that being a Christian pays for itself.

Nonetheless, several self-help projects in the meantime are running well: Jeffry now drives a motorbike taxi, just like Ate Donita's brother, Paulo. With approximately eight boys, we begin this week to slaughter chickens and to deliver them on order to houses or shacks free of charge. In Bagong Silang the Chicken Project is very successful; perhaps we can achieve something similar here. Two months ago, I founded a committee of Filipinos for the repairing and renovation of shacks that are falling down. In order to avoid jealousy, I chose four people from four different churches.

Upon reflection, I don't regret closing down our "Orphanage" in Bagong Silang. I understand that here everything is provisional, all of the small initiatives that we instituted, all of life, and it's also clear to me that the "Orphanage" could only be a transitional station for the teenagers who had grown older and who had to learn to stand on their own feet. But despite that, it makes me sad. Things grow close to one's heart.

I am supposed to conserve my energy. This is insanely difficult for me, but I'm simply too tired to be able to continue this way much longer. There is also a small wound on my shin bone that has not healed well in the last three months.

Today I read various facts about the eruption of Pinatubo, which they have more or less understood statistically: The volcano had engorged two and a half cubic miles of material and thereby lost 850 feet in height. The tropical thunder and rain that occurred over the region a little later caused approximately 8,000 houses to cave in because of the heavy ash-water-mixture that had fallen on the roofs. Over 800 people lost their lives. Hundreds of square miles of agricultural land became unusable. And here in the slum people fight their way through life, either as servants in the helping mode or as Filipino in survival mode.

I turn my thoughts to God and to the people in the chapel, to the shining eyes, to Jojie, who stopped dying and again awakened to life. And so I go to sleep.

Katja, the Temporary Missionary

Two days ago, we devout Christians were in the headlines. An attack on a Christian mission's ship took place in the harbor of Zamboanga, a city in the southern Philippines. Apparently it was perpetrated by fanatical Muslims. Two dead, thirty-two seriously injured people from sixteen countries.

I know that ship. It belongs to an American Evangelical Mission Association and is a kind of floating mission station and bookstore. The ship anchors somewhere, and the young Christians on board fan out into the streets of the city, sell Christian books and tracts, organize street theater, present films or seminars. Some go the marketplaces, to schools and prisons, some to conference rooms on-board ship. Whenever possible, they work together with local congregations. I appreciate this work and know that thousands of young people acquire worthwhile experience that will serve them their whole life long. The founder of this Mission Association is one of the exemplary models of my youth.

Last evening a member of the Swiss Embassy telephoned. Three Swiss women are among the wounded, and they are seeking Swiss nationals living in Manila who could visit them in the hospital. And so today, in the early afternoon, I am marching through the corridors of the Makati Medical Center (MMC) in the most modern business district of the capital with its skyscrapers with their shiny glass and steel facades.

Based on its reputation, the MMC is the best and also the most expensive private hospital in Manila. Just like a Swiss hospital, it carries the scent of disinfectant and cleanliness, not of urine and sweat, as the government hospitals in the northern part of the city where the corridors are dirty and full of patients. Well, alright, when they're injured and far from home, the young missionaries at least receive first-class medical care.

I step into a room and find myself opposite a surprised young woman named Katja. She appears pale and exhausted, but she is smiling. I learn that they had operated on her buttocks, back, neck, and head, but the worst seemed over. "They were able to remove some metal fragments. I still have two splinters in my head, in some dangerous places, with which the physicians aren't quite sure how to proceed."

Her head and neck position is unnaturally cramped. I assume that every motion causes her pain. I sit down and ask Katja how this could happen, and she tells me the story.

"We spent two wonderful weeks in Zamboanga. Many congregations and schools opened their doors and were pleased to work with us. The local government also seemed friendly and built a large stage directly in front of the government building. On the last evening, an "International Night" took place—an evening of entertainment with free admission. Because of a severe thunderstorm we had to move the program into the harbor's booking and clearing hall. We presented joyful folkloric offerings from the various countries of the world. Approximately 1,500 audience members from the city were present, and the atmosphere was very pleasant. After the presentations, a passionate evangelical sermon was given by one of the leaders. During this time, behind the stage, many people from the ship prayed for the event. And then suddenly two hand grenades flew onto the stage. One exploded approximately ten feet from me. Because of the force of the explosion, I was catapulted onto a colleague sitting next to me. In shock, I wobbled in the direction of the exit, but soon collapsed.

It was mad confusion, shards and blood everywhere. We were afraid and only wanted to get away!"

Katja paused. I ask her about her perception of this deed. She says, "I can forgive those who did this. I don't feel any hate. Naturally, I am sad. But why God allowed this, what good this will do, I don't know. Those are open questions."

Impressive.

On the way home I again tackle the basic question, why God allowed this. "Because we learn from this," or "God is not responsible for our messes," and other standard answers are not enough for me. Why does God allow poverty, degradation, hate, and bloodshed?

Of course, I create my own proverbial adage based on this incident. There is a southeast Asiatic city, approximately three times as large as Basel, in which at least one quarter of the population is Muslim and a considerable portion lives in great poverty. Then a ship arrives with a few hundred young people, beautiful, well-nourished people from rich, beautiful, well-nourished countries, who want to spread their faith, with many words and little help. After two or three weeks, they leave to return to their over abundance. What they leave behind are words, books, and poverty. This is how I assess the perception of at least a critical minority in this port city.

Surely, the young "missionaries" on the ship receive preparatory training in which they learn to approach other cultures and religions respectfully and with appropriate esteem. But for this it is not only necessary to receive training and have some interest in the social reality of the hosts, but rather to have *much* interest and also *much* time to enter into this reality and to learn to understand the language and society of these people, at least incrementally. Three weeks of talking should be preceded by three years of listening. Jesus of Nazareth lived in Palestine for thirty years before he began to heal and preach.

Those who would "missionize" people, without sharing a piece of their lives and seeking friendship, degrade those people to mission objects and the mission to a shared event. And I find this disrespectful in relation to the people as well as to the message of Jesus. For some Filipinos these young Amerikanos surely embody a large dose of presumption and know-all egoism.

One may not blame the young people on this ship. I don't consider Katja as lacking in respect or arrogant. She seems to me to be a fine young woman who operates according to the best of her knowledge and conscience. But she grew up—as did I—in a naïve First World.

The Fresh Breeze

Nobody in the neighborhood expected it, but Jojie is actually much better. Now and again he still spits blood, but I regularly bring him expensive medications that can cure a patient of tuberculosis under normal circumstances, provided that he takes them regularly for three to six months, and provided he doesn't die in the meantime, because of a hemorrhage, for example.

About one month ago, Jojie came strolling into our chapel on Sunday morning and reported that he had become a Christian and God had healed him. I had to smile because at that time he was still quite yellow in his face. But he was beaming. Since then, he regularly attended religious services, each time a little healthier. Recently he has been responsible for the community's cash from the Sunday collection.

As I stop by at Jojie's this morning with his medications, he shows me knife marks in the wood wall of his shack. And then he tells me what happened the night before last: "Each year on the same night in this part of Potrero, a kind of ritual murder occurs. Mostly a group of men get drunk and decide on a victim. It's always a man who in their view deserves to die for one reason or another. They then stab him. This time they wanted to kill Edwin.

Edwin is Jojie's nephew, an exceedingly fresh teenager, lacking in respect, who gives not only Jojie a lot of trouble. I met him a few days ago since he was visiting Jojie for several weeks.

"In any case, the men came after midnight. I realized immediately what was happening, stood in their way and screamed that they had to stab me first if they wanted my visitor. Then we withdrew into the house, step by step. Several of the men, enraged, stuck their knives in the closed door and the wall. Suddenly, however, they stopped and went away. It was the first time in years that no one had to die on this night. Thank God!"

A horrible situation brought to a close without unpleasantness. Was it by chance or a miracle? When I see Jojie's eyes, and his life that brought him the message of a loving God, I decide on behalf of a miracle, without question.

The next day I visit Navotas, the stilt-houses slum by the cemetery. The paths to the shacks appear more solid, since the bamboo stalks have been replaced with wooden boards with the help of contributions from Switzerland. The men have also built a kindergarten. Juliet, an experienced teacher and slum resident, oversees it. One can tell that she is originally from the upper middle-class.

When I arrive she leads me to the end of the settlement to a newly erected pole shack directly on the ocean front and says, "Our community built you a hut. We want you to live with us. It's also not as hot here as in the city. Can you feel the fresh breeze from the ocean?"

The thought is tempting and the invitation feels good—my presence is appreciated. But I have not received permission from the Servants team to move here. In Navotas, there would again be a need for survival training that would take up all of my time. Therefore, I decline. Juliet is disappointed but I promise her that I will visit once a week and stay overnight with them in the hut.

In the news that evening, the assault on the mission ship is a topic. The perpetrators belonged to Abu Sayyaf, an Islamic terror organization that is particularly active in the Muslim South of the Philippines. The reason for the deed makes me angry: Workers from the mission ship were invited to a discussion with Islamic students at a school. There, a young, eager Christian got it into his head to make a insensitive and stupid pronouncement that Mohammed was a liar.

Of course there was an outcry that pervaded the Muslim population. Abu Sayyaf knew how to use this for their own purposes—and the leader of the delegation had to apologize publicly for the pronouncement by the overly eager temporary missionary. So much for the topic "Respect and appreciation of the worth of other cultures."

It is already relatively late as I climb onto my plank-bed. Although I'm terribly tired, as all too often in the last months, I can't fall asleep right away. My thoughts center on and around Switzerland. Regula, Christian, and I have rented a house, our "Swiss House"—as a guesthouse as well as for "retreats" of all kinds. We were able to take over the furnished house at a very generous rental price from departing missionaries. Now we have six rooms in a quiet, clean location, and for that we are very grateful. We Swiss can spend time with one another and create a little Swiss ambience. How I have missed that!

Naturally, we three don't need such a large house only for administrative matters, meetings, and retreats. But late in the fall, Regina and Markus Meyer and their three children will join us. They too want to try living with the poor in the slum. A true challenge with three children! Regula, Christian, and I will provide them lodging in the first couple of weeks in our Swiss House and will support them as much as possible in their immersion into the world of poverty.

The next four weeks will be overwhelmingly Swiss: Sixteen friends from Germany and Switzerland are coming to visit. A few are considering the question if they might also want to join Servants. The others simply want to learn to know and better understand the life of the poor and our work here. I am looking forward with great pleasure to the weeks with these friends. A fresh breeze will waft through my life in the slum. Christine is her name.

If She Survives . . .

Today the Swiss group will arrive. We have planned their visit well: An introductory week in the Swiss House will mark the beginning, then two weeks with a slum family follows, and finally our "apprentices" will enjoy a couple of days to recover on Boracay, the vacation isle.

Finding slum families willing to be hosts for two weeks is the least of our problems. I saw to it that Christine would come to a family in Potrero, very near to me. Hardworking and amiable parents, eight children, the lodgings a damp and dark hole. If she survives this, she'll survive almost anything.

Christine retained the experiences of the first days by describing them in writing:

Frankfurt, August 24, 1991. My first flight to another part of the world! The jumbo jet is filled to capacity. We are sixteen Swiss and Germans who want to experience the work of Servants in Manila and the life of the inhabitants of the slum close up. I gave it a try, without hoping too much, to lodge with a slum family that possibly lives close to Chris. . . .

After our arrival in the Swiss House in a gated, guarded quarter, we had an Asian meal: roast chicken, rice, vegetables, bananas, and for dessert a conference with Regula, whose name here is Rachel, as well as with Christian Auer and with Chris. The latter informed us right away where we will be living. And what do you know—I am very close to him!

Monday. *The first visit to a poor quarter in the Frisco slum where Christian Auer lives. We are invited to eat by his host mother Aling Esther. Thereafter we "stroll" as a group through the small alleys: I have to take care not to step into the sewage or dog dirt below, or to bump my head on one of the slanted awnings above.*

It seems as if the people here live as in a camp: Fetch water, cook on the butane gas stove, wash the laundry in large plastic basins on the floor. I ask myself how they can do it, even wearing a lily-white T-shirt in the evening! They move about in the middle of the filth gracefully and with dignity. My admiration grows. We are impressed by the heartfelt and joyous demeanor of the people. I wonder what they think of us "tourists"?

Sunday, September 1. *Moving out of the Swiss House. The end of the days of grace in the sanctuary. Moving into the wilderness with Mother Alin Joy, Father Kuya Rolando and their eight children between one and fourteen-years-old. Here I have something ahead of me! The proximity to Chris is, to be sure, almost as exciting. Here he can test me relatively without problem as to my fitness for the slum. I will be living with ten people for two weeks in a partition of approximately six by eight feet with only a plank-bed . . . and with a nervous feeling in my stomach.*

Monday. *I slept together with two girls on the plank-bed. Or better said: I tried. It is narrow. It is hot. I hear rats constantly running over the tin roof. But at least I'm protected by a mosquito net. Chris got it for me. I showered in the smallest space, with a dipper and water out of a rain barrel. The shower is in the public alleyway of the slum and is used by numerous families. One can close oneself in with a lever, but everyone who wants to can watch me through the cracks. If I survive this. . . .*

For Chris's female neighbors, we visitors from Switzerland are a welcome change of pace. I don't understand a single word, but the way they laugh and chatter, I have the feeling that they're waiting for one of us Swiss women to pair off with Chris. The children are enthusiastic about my visit, and speak Tagalog to me without interruption. They read my every wish in my eyes; all of them treat me like a queen. And I can't give them anything at all. I feel disconcerted by so much hospitality.

Aling Joy and I go to the market together and buy crabs, fish, and meat. Everything is full of flies, it stinks horribly and I am glad when we return to the shack. It is unclear to me how I will be able to eat. Then I am amazed, however: Aling Joy cooks and fries the things a long time and her food tastes good.

On **Tuesday** *morning at 6:00 o'clock, some of us who "live" in Potrero meet with Chris. In a tiny room he has prepared breakfast rolls and hot chocolate for us. What a treat after all the rice! We don't have any quiet to talk: Neighbors come by constantly, ask about something, or sit down with us for a little while. Generally, Chris is on the go without interruption, on his way to all the projects that he oversees. Opportunities to chat arise now and then on the trips through the city. Slowly I realize happily that he wants to get to know me better. I am eager to see how he plans to do this, since one has hardly a single quiet minute here. To talk together* *alone near the slums would be a transgression against Asian culture and would aid and abet wild rumors.*

Friday, September 6. *At the evening program Chris says that I received a fax at the Swiss House that morning, and asks if I would like to read it tonight. First I decline. After the first five days in the slum, we are allowed to treat ourselves to a weekend at the Swiss House tomorrow anyway. But suddenly it occurs to me that we decided at home that my family should write only in an emergency. Is it possibly an emergency? Besides, it also occurs to me that Chris might drive me there. After the evening program I ask him if perhaps he wouldn't mind. . . .*

He drives me. On his motorcycle. Through half of Manila. That I really wouldn't have imagined. And I have the impression that he doesn't care, and I definitely don't either. How exciting, a motorcycle ride alone with Chris!

The emergency turns out not to be one: The fax contains only a lot of greeting from Basel, which is very embarrassing. Help! My dear family pursues me halfway around the world! But after this ride in the late evening, Chris's goodbye is very personal. I can't sleep for a long time because I'm so excited.

Christine goes about things in a good way. She is beautiful and smart and she knows exactly what she wants. As a grade school teacher, she teaches migrant children. Besides, she worked full-time for several years in the youth program of the CVJM. She really isn't easily shocked. Her unusual blue eyes glow, and her winning laughter is catching. If only we had more time! But I constantly race back and forth between Potrero, Bagong Silang, and Navotas.

This is the phase in which one doesn't really know if one has a connection or not. Presumably we have one, we just haven't spoken about it. In our travel group there are several single women, and I have the feeling that they sense something. In the group I try to act as impartial and discreet as possible, and Chris too doesn't give any indication.

Friday, September 13. *After barely two weeks, worthwhile friendships have developed between us and the inhabitants of Potrero, not least because we visitors helplessly entrusted ourselves to them. We were the weak, they the strong. Leave taking is difficult. Yesterday in my daily meditation I read in the Bible, "Share your bread with the hungry!" That I will take with me from my two apprentice weeks back to Switzerland.*

Before we leave we are allowed a couple of days on a paradisical island named Boracay. There we will rest, process what we have learned, and prepare for our return to Switzerland. We're all standing in front of the Swiss House, ready for the trip to the airport. How Christian always looks at me! Warm and lovingly. I enjoy it. Yes, we do have a connection. It is time to talk about it.

After a short flight and a two hour Jeepney ride through the jungle, we climb into a large fishing boat that brings us to our destination, a splendid sandy beach, in ten minutes. "Now one should be in love, then everything would be even more beautiful," one of the group remarks.

On the next day we take a sightseeing tour of the little island. And then in the afternoon, Christian whispers at a discreet moment: "We have to talk!" "Yes, I think so too," I respond, gratefully. Now I am shaking with excitement.

Actually, we manage to meet in the evening, alone, just the two of us, down on the beach sufficiently far away from the others. We sit close together in the snow-white sand of Boracay, holding hands, and gazing silently at the deep blue ocean. Christine is 28, I am 34. She comes from the protected milieu of a typical small middle-class family, I from an apartment in public housing, inhabited by a laborer's family of eight. She is more of an introverted thinker, I am extroverted and spontaneous, a man of feeling through and through.

We have only five days left. Then I fly back. Somewhat crazy, under these circumstances, to talk about an enduring relationship. But that's exactly what I want. Otherwise I won't be able to bring this man to the point of coming to Switzerland.

At some point, the first words begin to slip out. About our love. About doubts and hopes. She lives in Basel. I live in Manila. Will our young love be steadfast despite harsh reality? I am torn hither and yon.

After this romantic beginning under palm trees and the sound of the waves, many lonely months lie before us in which we will have to satisfy ourselves writing letters. But we feel deep within us: We belong together!

More Swiss, Less Slum

New Year 1992—unbelievable how time flies! Christine and I have written letter after letter to one another in the last four months. Much has happened:

to the people in our projects, to Christine, to me. Most important, since a few days ago, I no longer live in my small partition in Potrero with Ate Donita, but rather in the Swiss House. This is certainly less slum and more Swiss, but does not contain as much Swiss as I would like.

These almost sentimental feelings for home are foreign to me. Is it because of age, because of the distance from Christine, or because of the fatigue that I feel more often than before? In the last years I have indeed undertaken too much, throwing myself into one project after the other, have initiated things, built them up.... And now I find myself feeling somewhat "injured."

For example, Edwin, who was saved from a ritual murder by the intercession of his Uncle Jojie—this Edwin stole from his brave uncle, the cashier of our Potrero church, the congregation's cash box and fled. One can't really grasp it. I have a different conception of the course of events. The fact that the congregation that developed parallel to the "Orphanage" in Bagong Silang has had numerous changes in pastoral leadership is on my mind. Earlier such situations did not wound my perception of the world and humanity in the least. And today?

Today, actually, not really. God is here. But I'm simply tired, and my resistance is low. I think of Rob and Lorraine, how they left Bagong Silang abruptly almost two and a half years ago, and returned to New Zealand, fully exhausted. My move into the Swiss House is probably wise. Thank God Regula and Christian are here, and will move to Potrero, where they will join Pastor Pepe, the congregation leadership and others, in overseeing the ministry.

Sometimes I fear that everything will deflate while I'm away, because so much has arisen only because of my own initiative and activism. I hope very much that a great deal of what I have done will prove to be long lasting. With this, I must rely on God.

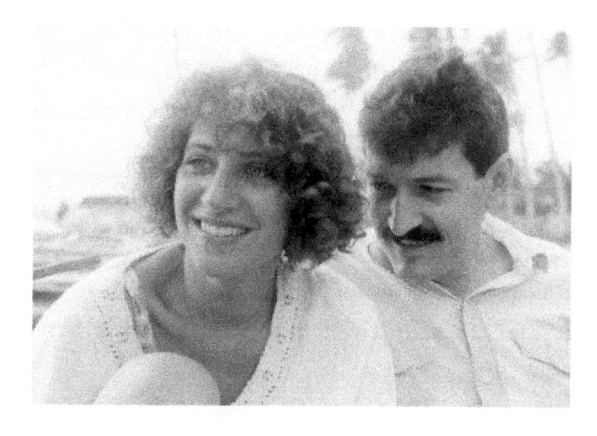

After this romantic beginning under the palms, a few lonely months lay before us ...

These months in the Swiss House make my leave taking easier. In spring or summer I will return to Switzerland. I am drawn by Christine. I must and want to know her better, and I must be clear myself whether I am capable and ready for a committed relationship, for a marriage. I am not a simple man, and if I were Christine, I would think twice about marrying me. But I think that Christine knows what she's in for with me.

Interim Balance

It's almost time. Next week I fly home to Switzerland. Then I will have spent almost four years in Manila, from June 1988 until April 1992. My emotional world is in turmoil when I see what has and what hasn't happened in the few months since my move into the Swiss House.

The ex-gangster Boboy disappeared again some time ago. Someone saw him a few weeks ago with a revolver. A few days ago I visited Boboy's relatives who told me he had lovingly cared for his sick father for a number of weeks. Having been reconciled with God, he himself then died of tuberculosis. Can that be true? It could be that they made up the story in order to comfort me, in Asian style.

The ex-gangster Rico from the graveyard slum has been successful on his path away from criminality, earns an income for himself and his family with his sandal manufactory and is true, along with his family, to the Potrero Congregation. Wouldn't you know, he, with whom I made the "money for faith" deal, seems to be one of my "good shots." God certainly has a dry sense of humor.

The ex-gangster Romeo, on whose land the chapel in Potrero stands, was actually supposed to awaken an auto body shop to new life, with a larger grant from the Community Committee. The project seemed very promising. But then, the project money "disappeared," and Romeo began to drink again and to abuse his wife and children. My stomach almost turns over. Numerous men had counted on finding jobs in the workshop.

The ex-gangster Paulo, Ate Donita's brother, works hard as a motorcycle-taxi driver in order to pay for his motor bike, and is active in the leadership of the congregation in Potrero.

Jojie's face finally has lost its yellow cast entirely. He is a faithful soul and an active member of the congregation leadership in Potrero, together with Pastor Pepe, Ate Donita, and other devoted people.

The chicken project with the younger men proved to be unsuccessful in comparison to Bagong Silang. The lack of discipline of the young men drives me to despair. Some can't add, others come late to work, after a sale, money in the cash register goes missing, spoiled and inadequately cleaned chickens are delivered to clients—terrible! We would need to institute a remedial residential community here, to teach the boys how to live life—slowly, steadily, and with much, much patience. Some miracles apparently take time.

The kindergarten in the cemetery slum in Navotas runs well, the Bible Circle with Ate Juliet is regularly attended by Christian Auer and often also by Pastor Pepe.

The job creation projects, the building of the fountain with the cooperatives, the sponsorship program in Bagong Silang are all continuing without me, thank God! The same holds true for the small clinic, the kindergarten, the nutrition project, and the congregation at the chapel. I hope that after the change in pastors, peace will prevail. Darwin, a fine, experienced Filipino pastor, is in the process of taking over the leadership responsibilities.

The fact that our "Orphanage" is now closed because Albert was overcome by the problems of the boys and withdrew from the small congregation due to theological differences, pains me. I was very attached to those boys.

The chemistry between the leadership of Servants and me is currently not aligned. I am accused of doing too much too soon, that I worked too often with material help and overwhelmed the people, so that new problems ensued. This probably contains a kernel of truth. That I jumped into the work too vigorously is apparent in my fatigue. But when I look at each case, each story unto itself: What would have been the alternative? Hunger, misery, and a life of crime.

To do nothing and watch is also no solution. When one wants to change things, mistakes will be made. The work with the poor will always be accompanied by lack of success. Whoever is not prepared for that should remain in the worthy state of contemplation of a safe life. Despite all the setbacks, many people received help in these four years. This certainty crystallizes like a great surprise in me, and I won't let it be taken away.

I am overjoyed about the educated Filipinos from the middle-class who have decided to live with the poor. Three weeks ago, Dorie Morden actually left her quiet, large family home in the residential area of the wealthy and now lives with her also well-to-do girlfriend in a very modest brick shack, under a tin roof in a suburban slum!

And Jesse Sarol, my excellent language teacher and friend since my time in Bagong Barrio has been living for some time with Lenny and her three children in the Frisco slum. A few days ago, he passed his exit exams in linguistics, with honors. He was asked whether he wouldn't like to teach at a college. But he has heard the call from God to offer his life in the service of the poor.

In the small personal job creation projects for one-time criminals there are a few that still remain, others that do not. It's quite possible that most of them will whither away sooner or later. But for the first one or two years, they were very important, not only as a source for income, but also as a practice field for diligence, discipline, and honesty.

My luggage is packed. I am flying home. Grateful, but without assurance which direction my friends here will pursue in the long term. And only with presentiments how it could continue in Switzerland. I'm looking forward to Christine. To a couple of great mountain expeditions with my friend Urs Mayer—maybe Christine will come with us? And to slices of crème torte from the Migros supermarket with real fresh filtered coffee.

Romance is Sometimes Not Enough

I have a demanding winter behind me. A full curriculum as a teacher, and added to that the youth group, the church leadership, and much more. Plus there were the five months of waiting and dreaming about a man whom I hardly know. But now it is spring and Christian is landing in Switzerland. How often I have imagined this reunion . . . hopeful, rapt, and also somewhat anxiously tense.

A few of Christian's many friends ride with me to the airport at Zürich-Kloten. Fortunately I am not alone. To me, Christian is actually still a stranger. And then I see him in the arrival hall: A tired, handsome man, tanned by the sun. We wrote letters and faxes, sketching out the next few months, and then making a concrete plan; for example, where he will live and seek work. Now the time together begins.

Three years, London; four years, Manila. It's incredible how much Switzerland has changed in the seven years since 1985. Vivid violet and light green appear at the moment to be the actual modish colors of choice—they glow in my direction from hair clips, bicycles, and the jogging shorts of aging gentlemen.

The prosperity in Switzerland hasn't changed, but it hits me in the face with force nevertheless. Already during my first stroll through the streets of my native city, Basel, I feel as if I've been transported into an oversize automobile showroom. Unprotected and as a matter of course, the newest models from the world market stand at the curb, freshly polished and in meticulous condition. And although many citizens apparently own cars, every second one also keeps a luxurious mountain or city bike. Environmental protection has definitely become a topic; a luxury that only the rich can afford. And in the following summer months I notice in amazement that people romp and swim in the once dirty River Rhine.

As I climb down the long stairs in the historical inner city from *Steinebachgässli* down to the shopping street *Steinen*, I am surprised about another reality in Switzerland: There is trash here, and it smells of urine. Hardly a spot on the walls and battlements is not smeared with graffiti. They give expression to the frustration and obscenities of a generation that hungers for meaning and life.

The time together is meted out in short intervals. Right away there is a three-week course for people from Europe who would like to travel to Asia with Servants. Christian is the interpreter, travel guide, and organizer—and I am his hanger on. Between all the activities we nonetheless find the time to talk about our relationship and to forge plans. I have the impression that Christian's decision for a committed relationship is difficult for him. Our conversations are serious and romance sometimes falls short. It is Christian's fight between "I will," and "can I do it?" I myself am in love and naturally convinced that we can do it. And I am without worries. That helps me, at least.

Step by step I feel restored in my familiar cultural milieu. Fortunately, I have a lot to help me: for example cheese, Swiss chocolate, or fresh milk. There is as much of everything as the heart desires, or as my still sensitive stomach can stand. The "Danish Cup" in the ice cream parlor, with a fresh evening breeze, is extremely helpful in settling in; or, a spontaneous rock climbing party over the familiar limestone cliffs in the woods above Dornach, in the "Tüflete," together with Christine.

Today we went walking with my parents on the "Trogenhorn" in the Bernese Highlands. On the path into the valley we let the cat out of the bag: We want to become engaged. Christian and I will quickly buy rings tomorrow in Thun and then meet his mother and my parents to celebrate.

We find out the next day that one can't buy rings quickly. Two weeks until delivery appears to be normal. So we don't bother with the rings and drive to the lakeside resort in Thun to swim and to rest. That is, I swim, Christian rests. He finds water temperatures under 85 degrees too cold for swimming.

We go to the Migros Restaurant for lunch. There we have a further serious discussion: Christian admits his hesitation and I speak about my wishes and expectations of a relationship with him. We are absolutely honest and lay all our cards on the table. That pleases me. We now know what we're in for. Afterwards, Christian buys champagne, roses, and a cake, and we drive to the vacation house in Heimenschwand, where my parents and Christian's mother are waiting. It is a lovely evening with champagne and cake and without rings. What a lucky girl I am to be engaged to Christian Schneider!

Loving Christine is like a new morning in my life, a new sunny day. The obligation of our engagement worries me, however. Will the founding of a family mean my leaving Manila behind forever? A distasteful thought. Manila gave me a wealth of gifts in new friends and experiences. I feel something of the privilege of having become a part of another culture and language. On the other hand, I am tired, disillusioned, injured because of personal failure and the failure of others. The suffering and the grief of the poor have become a part of my own inner disposition. I have the feeling that the powerlessness of the poor and the insight that I can't change their suffering on the whole, have engendered an inner vulnerability in me. Peculiar. And: I have become conscious of my own powerlessness.

At the same time, through these experiences I have encountered God in new ways. I have recognized him in the faces of people, in their laughter, their tears, their rage, their life. I have experienced his presence in the life of communities as hardly ever before. I want to hold fast to the joyful realization of how hope awakened can create change. That joy should become my incentive in the coming years.

I have a job as a nurse in a community healthcare center. Besides this, from the first day forward, I am naturally again immersed in the life of the church with all its facets and all my friendships. Church congregations and schools invite me to tell them about my experiences in the slums. I discover that my lectures help me to keep my insights and memories fresh and to process them. When I tell stories about Bagong Silang and Potrero, I often find myself near tears. The insane contrast between Asian slum life and Swiss prosperity is so unjust that it hurts.

I sit here in 95 degree heat in the Boboli Gardens in Florence. My sister Judith and I have had a fun and relaxing time here on vacation. On the day after tomorrow

I will be in Basel again and perhaps on the same day will talk to Christian about planning our wedding: We're getting married in three months!

We will live in Christian's one-and-a-half room apartment, which he has furnished with furniture and dishes from the second-hand shop. A real challenge to my desire for an aesthetically pleasing interior décor. For years I have been sharing a flat and would very much like to have a whole furnished apartment, and now this! We will live with each other in one room, with a folding wall between bed and living room, which is the kitchen and dining room at the same time. The advantage is that we aren't establishing ourselves too permanently, in case of a new journey abroad with Servants.

A Challenging Entry into a Dynamic Life

I have been married to Christian for three weeks—Christine Schneider-Tanner! The days could not have been busier and more intense. The preparations, the celebration with almost three-hundred people from the whole world over, including the Philippines. All this was only possible thanks to our families and our friends in Basel. It was overwhelming!

After the wedding Christian had a surprise for me: three days free for a winter trip into the Swiss Alps. Only the two of us. I enjoyed these days to the utmost, knowing full well that upon our return, the first thing on the program would be a tour of Switzerland with the friends from the Philippines as well as visits to Christian's relatives and mission friends. For me, as an introverted person with a certain need for private time, this was a challenging entry into a dynamic life.

We didn't buy any new furniture. Why would we? Our apartment consists of only one and a half rooms. Besides, we want to keep the possibility open to be able to leave Switzerland one of these days with just the most necessary items. We haven't really discussed this in detail, but it's clear to both of us that we want to keep this prospect open. Heavy furniture, thick carpets, or a luxurious car should not stand in the way of a quick exit.

Christian tries very hard to postpone the thought of a return to Manila in the near future. We need some time to become used to a life together and to become a family. Nevertheless, Manila is always present since Christian travels so much to give lectures. Fundraising is a part of it, since the projects are supposed to continue.

I have reduced my work as a teacher considerably. In order to have some time together with Chris despite all of his activities, I gave up long-standing commitments such as the youth program and the church leadership. Is this really good for me? Perhaps, in spite of everything, I should retain a piece of my own life. But it's not so easy. If I want to be with him, I have to join him in his activities most of the time.

Christian can move people, carry them along with him. He looks attractive and athletic, makes a good impression, is empathetic and becomes engaged with everyone who knocks on his door. His life is full of people, and sometimes I fear being just one of the many. But most of the time it's simply exciting and nice to travel with him!

Being married is wonderful, but definitely not an ongoing honeymoon. Pleasant and difficult moments alternate as one probes one another's hopes and possibilities and has to adapt in many instances. This is an enormous challenge for two individuals who have been single for a long time. Not to expect one's partner to be responsible for one's happiness or unhappiness—and not to accept responsibility for the happiness or unhappiness of one's partner has to be learned. One has to be careful about expectations. Fortunately, experienced married couples stand with us as advisers and friends.

Something is different. My body is somehow not the same. First a suspicion. Then certainty. Then an incredible joy: I am pregnant! I can't quite grasp it! Pregnant already! When I tell Christian, he is also overjoyed. For both of us, it's a miracle. I am thirty, Christian is thirty-six; we hoped for a child soon . . . and now we're racing at top speed from marriage to a family.

Naturally I enjoy Christian's concern about me. I have his undivided attention, which feels good! Despite the uncertain future, I soon give in to the inclination toward nest building. Torn between admiration and amusement, Christian watches me as I shop, sew for hours, and move the furniture around—in which the variations in placement are limited.

And then there are these thoughts again, the Manila thoughts. In case we were to leave again, a sensible point in time would be around the first birthday of our child. Good that we have some time until then. Imagining leaving Switzerland with a child is much more difficult. At first I keep my thoughts to myself, because once I give Christian my okay for the Philippines, there's no taking it back. I know how much he wants to live in his second home again.

A Difficult Birth

The birth was to have taken place almost two weeks ago. Our child is not concerned about that. Already so headstrong; apparently takes after Christian. . . . I climb with Christian through the Jura, our forested hills, cheerfully pant up and down the stairways while in the meantime I can easily rest my coffee cup on my stomach. The child inside seems unperturbed.

Christian and I really do have different notions and inclinations, actually in almost every respect. In these circumstances, agreeing on the name for a child can be as taxing as our wandering through the Jura. Finally, we solve the problem pragmatically, as so often: He will choose the name if it's a boy, and I will choose if it's a girl.

It is the middle of the night, and Christine's water breaks. I am completely beside myself. Carefully I put Christine into the car and drive her to the Bruderholz Hospital. The people there seem much too calm and sleepy. Hey, my wife has an enormous stomach and is in considerable pain, and our little one is going to stick its head out any minute—get a move on!

My agitation makes little difference; the team remains relatively relaxed. Then the long wait begins. Hours and hours. The opening of the uterus simply doesn't want to dilate sufficiently. The labor pains are strong and keep coming with undiminished pain. Christine is suffering. My respect for her and all mothers of the world rises to the immeasurable. Pushing, again and again. The nurse stimulates. I sweat under a shower cap and mask. Christine can't do it anymore; she is totally worn out and wants to give up. Nothing is moving.

Now the birthing staff also seems nervous. "We have to call the Chief," one of the nurses whispers into my ear. "The heartbeat of the child is becoming weaker."

I am afraid. What did I cause? The child is too low for a Caesarean section, and it can't go back again. God in Heaven!

The Chief physician seems calm and asks me if I want to stay. Of course! "Don't worry. We'll get it out with forceps."

I clasp Christine's hand. They cut, and the blood flows like crazy; then a couple of practiced motions, a visibly forceful gesture by the Chief—and then he twists a dark something three times around its own axis and counts loudly as he twists: "Once, twice, three times the umbilical cord around the neck." My breath stops, but the doctor laughs: "The little one is fine." He lays the little something on a green towel. It actually moves and slowly color appears in the little face. Hallelujah! I'm a father!

With our child we now have a great mutual assignment. Sometimes our strength almost runs out. When Isabel suffers with stomach cramps and cries for hours, we take turns carrying her around the living room. Sometimes around midnight, Christian packs her into the car and drives her around until she is finally exhausted and falls asleep.

During the day I'm usually at home alone with her. Isabel doesn't want anyone but me. Every two hours she wants to eat; I feel tied down and lonely. For the first time in my marriage, I long to have people around me.

It occurs to me how uncomplicated it seemed in Manila to have a baby. In the slums the whole neighborhood helps to raise a child. I would not only learn the language and the life, but also with a baby I would have a prescribed role and duty. Actually, we're supposed to leave for the Philippines as a family in the near future. Not too many Swiss can imagine doing something like this. We can. Africa would interest me more, actually, but Christian knows the language and culture of the Philippines. It really makes sense for us to go to Manila.

Today, Christine thought aloud, how it would be to live in the slum. That is like a starting shot! Finally. A new chapter. In Manila, we will need the protection and the support of a team. We are not solitary warriors, so we will either move under the roof of the Servants in Manila again, or structure our life there under the leadership of Filipino NGO's or Philippine church communities. I have to go to Manila soon to resolve these questions.

Yesterday Volker Heitz and Christian returned from Manila. The Servants there are prepared to support us and to become our new family, he says. The Servants in Switzerland will take care of the organizational issues here in Basel. Next week Christian will write the resignation letter for his employers and give notice on our apartment.

Everything is moving almost too quickly for me. Now that our departure has become so concrete and well-known, I almost panic from time to time: Do I really want to do this? Fortunately, I don't get to the point of indulging my feelings. Each week we go a step further: Notification at the Residence Bureau; writing letters to all our acquaintances; preparing goodbye parties. How Christian manages to do all this!

Departure moves closer. From Switzerland. From our parents, who are here for us. From my sister, who has taken everything about the baby better than I have and with whom I get along so well. From my brother, who loves and cherishes us. A great relief for us is that despite heavy hearts, our families fully support our plans. Nonetheless, I anticipate the forthcoming leave taking with great sorrow.

I have become aware of the fact that Christine finds the parting with friends and relatives far more difficult than I do. I expect a lot of her. But fortunately, we have the same desire. For me, the joyful anticipation of the unknown and the reunion with old friends in Manila prevails!

I take full advantage of every moment with my near and dear now. Isabel is being spoiled and coddled by everyone. With my sister Judith and our two babies, I attend a Mother-Baby Week in Tessin, the Italian part of Switzerland. On Thursday the husband of the course leader appears and tells us that at home, while praying, he had a sort of vision in which he saw a strong, warm tropical rain pouring down on a mother, as a symbol of blessings and renewal. Everyone agrees that this image must apply to me, so close to departure to a tropical land. This impression will surely accompany me and provide comfort in certain situations.

Many friends and relatives attended the official going-away party sponsored by our congregation in Basel. There is so much support! As representatives of so many people in Switzerland and Germany, we go to the poor. . . .

We are standing in the train station in Basel. There is no going back now. My father-in-law, René, joins us on the train that will take us to the Zurich airport. He wants to take advantage of every last minute. We embrace each other. René's eyes are moist and he trembles, and I could also begin sobbing. What I demand of him and Alice! I am taking away their daughter and granddaughter and am leading them into a dangerous world. But they and also my own aged mother have supported us in the preparations in every possible way. I did not notice a single reproachful word or glance. What magnanimity!

It is two years and four months since my arrival in Switzerland. Now, on October 8, 1994, I am sitting in a jumbo jet on the runway of the Zurich airport and am returning to Manila—with a wife and a little daughter. How really crazy all of this seems!

Letters from Manila

October 11, 1994. Hello, my dear ones, on our second day in the Phillipines. We just now returned from a long, hot, and dusty ride through the city. Chris and Isabel are making a quick visit to a Filipino friend, a dentist, and I am enjoying a restful moment after a pleasant shower. I feel a little better than yesterday, when I was totally limp from jet lag and the heat. And this is supposed to be the "cool" time of year! At night, because of the time difference, we lay awake for hours. Isabel, too, needs a little calming syrup when she wakes up at 2:00 a.m. That helped us on the plane—she slept soundly!

We went to the Swiss Embassy to secure a visa for three years and could then pick up our baggage that we sent by air freight. We had "good luck": The procedure took only two hours instead of a half day, because we found the right office on the first try. Nonetheless, Chris ran from one staff member to another about twenty times and gathered stamps on his freight papers.

To make the four-hour ride through the city more pleasant, we took a taxi. This is very cost effective here and cool, with air conditioning. Also all supermarkets are air conditioned. One continuously moves between the cool temperatures inside and the heat outside. Isabel is amused by all this. She sweats all day long, but is content and happy. Everywhere, she is admired, pinched, smiled at, and she enjoys it. She is not afraid of the people, quite the opposite: She sometimes smiles back and is rarely shy.

As we drove through the twelve- to sixteen-lane streets today, we became newly aware of how many people here live under miserable circumstances, in a city where there is also much luxury. The differences between rich and poor are terribly crass. An entire family stands on the highway—in unspeakable dirt and stench. The little children jump between the half-standing, half-moving cars, to sell chewing gum or to beg for money. And right next door there is a giant "Shopping Temple," with a paradisical children's playground and everything that one can imagine.

Naturally, we will always live in both worlds in order to actually endure this. But we will share a great part of our lives here with the poor, and I look forward to it, even though I see difficult times coming in my direction.

Soon our Philippine cook at the Servants house will have supper ready. Together with the couple that manages the house and a few missionaries, we will sit at the table and most certainly eat rice and a side dish of vegetables and meat or fish. Today at noon, we were in one of the many fast food restaurants, where one can eat good meals. We're doing very well!

My dear ones, I wish that you could experience everything here with us. It is a totally different life! I am already more optimistic than I was yesterday. When one first arrives, one thinks that one will not be able to stand it here in this city. But one gets used to everything new very quickly.

See you soon, Your Christine

October 13, 1994. *Dear Ones, we're doing very well after this first week in the Philippines. We're looking for a place to live in one of the slums.*

Today I also experienced the first tropical rain. Within a quarter hour the street was flooded. The Filipinos watched without comprehending, as we, with Isabel, ran laughing and squealing through the rain. They believe ardently that one becomes sick by standing in the rain without an umbrella or head cover.

What is different about our daily life here? Lots of things! Everything is furnished more simply, even here in the Servants house. The windows are always open, without a ventilator nothing works, one constantly drinks cold water, one eats mostly toasted bread, rice, vegetables, and fish. One has to put everything away very securely because of the ants and rats—and one constantly needs a cloth, in order to wipe off the sweat. Sometimes the electricity fails, or the water stops running. Then one has to be flexible.

Love, Your Christine

October 21, 1994. *Dear Ones, two weeks in Manila—and I feel completely at home. That will most likely change again, when I experience the usual culture shock, namely then when everything is no longer new and exciting, but becomes troublesome, unpleasant, and difficult. At the moment, however, everything is going extremely well. Isabel has also become accustomed to the new climate and people to the best possible degree. Life as a part of the greater family here in the Servants house has many advantages. There are always a few missionaries on hand who are taking a break or working in the office. The children entertain one another, and one is never alone. We have just returned from a five-day retreat with the Servants team: five families with ten children, the caretaker couple, our Philippine cook, Aida, and six single people. We drove five hours beyond Manila, to a paradisical place: a giant area full of palm trees with swimming pool and waterslide . . . not bad, is it? One pays less than 10 franks per day (6 US dollars) including all meals.*

In the morning for three to four hours, the children were cared for, and we had Bible discussions, exchange of ideas, and prayers for one another. It was a stirring, lively situation! People who live with the poor carry a great deal of need and sorrow personally. One notices that in the missionaries. God gave us impressions and

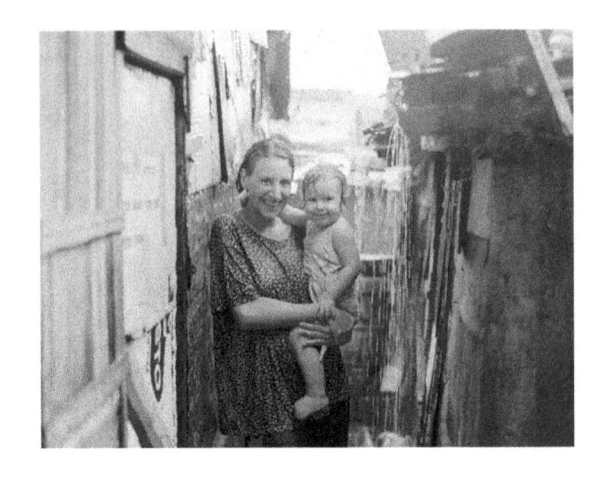

The Filipinos looked on in puzzlement as we, with Isabel, ran through the rain laughing and squealing.

impulses that helped and comforted. The time together allowed us to become a part of the family.

We continue to investigate slums in which we could live. Then I will also have my first Tagalog lesson.

Love, Christine

October 25, 1994, 8:00 p.m. *Dear Ones, we are so happy that in two weeks we will be able to move into our little slum house. We will live in the middle of ten to fifteen slum shacks, that are all built attached to one another. This "superstructure" is not bigger than a single-family house in Switzerland, but shelters about seventy people. On the other side of each of our plywood walls one or more families make their home. This Friday the carpenters from the slum quarter will begin to build a second floor onto the one-story house so that we can have a second room that will give us at least a little privacy. The lower floor will be finished with raw bricks; the second story is to be constructed of palm wood and plywood.*

The rent for this space amounts to 125 Swiss francs per month (79 US dollars). This lodging opportunity is a gift for us. Everything happened so easily and so quickly. Through a Filipino friend, Joshua, who also lives in the same superstructure, we met the owner of our shack. They are friendly people who are happy that we will move near them. The slum lies directly near a government building. A city park, the language school, and a wealthy quarter with swimming pool are also nearby. We have the impression that this will be an easy beginning before we perhaps move into a worse quarter, of which there are more than enough in Manila.

Last Sunday, a Filipino pastor took us to the famous "Smokey Mountain," a giant mountain of trash near to the harbor quarter. We were shocked by what we saw. One can hardly imagine it: Thousands of people and children, who crawl over the rubble. Stench, smog, smoke, and waste! Five- and six-year-old children go barefoot through the rubbish, some in flip-flops. They carry the garbage away in heavy baskets on their backs and sell it.

Our new friend, Joshua, has been living with these people voluntarily for seven years already. He lives in our neighborhood only temporarily and in phases, because he studies theology nearby. It certainly would have taken a great deal of self-control for me to get out of the car there, not to mention living there!

Love, Your Christine

November 6, 1994. Next Saturday we finally move into our little house. For the last three days we've had a visitor from Basel, Urs Mayer. He is helping us with furnishing and would like to stay for a few days thereafter and live in another slum. Urs brought us all kinds of delicious gifts; it was like Christmas!

This week we're buying the furniture for our little house. I find this very tiring—much driving around, searching, and bargaining. We're going to have very little room. The view from the second floor is actually very nice: A green lawn, a few trees, and in the distance a tall monument. Isabel is healthy, but has quite a few mosquito bites. We rub her with a strong lotion a few times a day. Yes, this is now part of life.

The weight of our one-year-old actually hangs mostly on me, literally, since one carries her practically everywhere. That is very hard on one's back. To take a buggy in the Jeepney is very awkward. We have taken various lovely day trips, however, to vary the everyday experience and to visit friends.

Three times a week I sit with my language helper, Jessica, and develop short stories about our family and daily events with her, which she then speaks into a recorder in Tagalog. Subsequently, I try to memorize these sentences. Then I stroll around the slum and say them to every conceivable neighbor, be they children, women doing laundry, or, now and then, also men who are sitting together and chatting or drinking beer. Of course, they laugh at me, because I still make many mistakes, but the neighbors are exceedingly proud and happy that they can teach me something. Later, at the language school, I will learn the grammar. Chris will refresh and deepen his language skills two mornings per week.

There are almost no foreigners who speak Tagalog. Filipinos are always immeasurably astonished when they hear Chris speaking in their language. Particularly since the Philippines were under foreign rule for so long (Spanish, American, Japanese). I find it is offensive when foreigners work with them and don't take the *trouble to learn their language. Without Tagalog, conversations always remain just small talk.*

With the move into our slum house, normal life will finally begin. We heartily hope that we will succeed in finding a good, healthy routine in which learning the language, the household, Isabel, the time we spend together and with God, the contacts with Switzerland, and also personal rest and leisure time will not fall short. All three of us have varying needs. To bring them all under one umbrella is challenging! Our heartfelt thanks for your prayers!
Christine

Beginnings in the NIA Slum

We have finally moved into our newly renovated shack. On the lower level the walls are made of cinder blocks, square footage of 13 x 12.5 feet, comprising cooking niche and bath/toilet. On the upper level we have 0.12 inch thick plywood and a corrugated tin roof. Our space is about three times the size as that of most Filipino families, which are also five to six persons larger than ours on the average.

First we filled the half-inch holes in the thin plywood, through which we could otherwise see directly into the living and sleeping quarters of the neighbors. The houses here are built unsystematically into and over one another.

Our shack belongs to Amy and Benjie, the parents of our neighboring family. They are industrious and upstanding, and we can really trust them. They watch over our Isabel whenever we need time to study, work, or rest. Amy maintains a little "Sari-Sari," a kind of general store, directly on the corner. Benjie drives a motorcycle taxi with a sidecar. The two are not only a two-income family, but actually three-income earners. They collect rent for an illegal slum apartment, namely ours! Strictly speaking, all slum dwellings are illegal to be sure.

Amy and Benjie have two boys and wish to have a daughter. They are crazy about our little Isabel, with her blond locks. Their four-year-old boy also seems overjoyed about "his" younger sister. When Isabel falls asleep in the evening on the floor of Amy's shack, next to the sleeping boys and the two dogs, also sleeping, nicely bedded down in pillows, we let her spend the night there. Isabel enjoys being together with the other children; she feels totally safe.

Joshua introduced us to the neighborhood, and thereby our arrival was much facilitated. As we moved in, he delivered the traditional house blessing.

For all the curious neighbors and onlookers, there were some sweet rolls, cola, and orange juice.

The NIA slum where we live takes its name from a gigantic government building complex next door, the "National Irrigation Authority." At the back the slum is sealed off by a small wall, a guarded empty field, a street, and finally by a thirteen-foot-high electrical fence with a deep pitfall. The Philippine National Bank, in which the gold of the country is stored and the Philippine money is printed, is hidden behind this. On another side, an open wastewater canal bounds our area. I estimate that NIA has about a thousand slum shacks—a rather small settlement of the poor.

The first days are boisterous. Here it's almost continually as loud as in a lively Swiss schoolyard. We are immersed in a changing bath of strong, vaporous odors: sometimes sweat and feces, then roasted fish, gasoline, smoke from a wood fire, beer and cigarettes, and in between completely foreign, disgustingly acrid smells the origin of which we can only imagine. Then this unpleasant, stinking wastewater trough running alongside of our shack, which we can't avoid since it is at the same time the only, barely two foot wide path to our home. And the aggressive mosquitoes...

Some slum dwellers, without a doubt, perceive us as a provocation. Many have grown accustomed to their role as victims and try to gain advantage thereby. With us that doesn't work, since we don't fit into the accepted separation of roles. We are not the rich white helpers, but rather the indigent. Although I have four years of slum experience, which I try to hide, these four years are by no means enough to prevent overweening demand and offense.

Altogether the atmosphere in our slum quarter is friendly. But sometimes the sparks fly nonetheless. Poverty and the cramped next to, on top of, and over one another seems to make the people aggressive. Three days ago, with approximately 40 other people, we squeezed ourselves onto the narrow wood benches in the little chapel not far from our shack. Also "present" at the service was a dead person. Next to the wall, lying in a coffin, was the corpse of an eighteen-year-old, who had been shot in a fight several shacks' distance from us. The gunman, the husband of a member of the congregation, subsequently disappeared.

Yesterday, at midnight, all hell broke loose in the adjacent shack—cursing, arguing, and it sounded as if someone was destroying the shack. I was afraid the fight had something to do with us. Did we give preferential treatment to someone during the building process? Jealousy can become an existential problem among the poor. We prayed for protection for us all. This morning we learned that while building a wooden stair, one neighbor stole some space from another. The latter drank some courage last night, and tore down the new stairway.

There is also friction between Christine and me. Stress erodes the power of resistance. The smallest things provide a reason for an unpleasant tenor between us. I am glad that my friend Urs Mayer is here! He helps me to better understand Christine's perception of things, since it seems that I, with my experience in the slum, am somewhat of a know-it-all. . . . In the meantime it's become clear to me that it can't be as before, to live on the same social level as our neighbors, particularly as pertains to our living arrangements. I have to concern myself more than before to assure that we as a family endure living in the slum for an extended period of time.

Letters from Manila

December 8, 1994. *Dear Ones, Urs leaves this afternoon! He has become sick, presumably it's typhoid fever. It could be that during a half-marathon he got some dirty water at a water station. Don't worry. Urs brought us a brand new Katadyn water filter and we drink this water exclusively!*

I have caught a really bad throat infection and am only slowly getting better. The antibiotics here are not the same as those in Switzerland. Isabel has two new teeth coming in and suffers a lot. She also has a lot of diarrhea and is cranky. Otherwise, she's doing fine, however. She spends a lot of time at the neighbors', and they take care of her so that we can learn the language. Since we live so close to the neighbors, we naturally hear everything, and they hear us. Sometimes I don't even

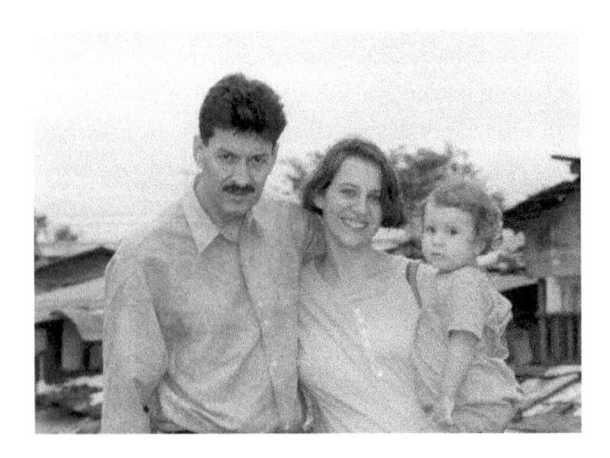

End of 1994: The first weeks in NIA. Fortunately, we don't yet know everything that will befall us!

know if a noise has come from our shack or from next door. Actually, in Tagalog, the "neighbor house" is "kapitbahay," literally translated: "Houses that embrace."

I have quickly gotten used to having little privacy. Nevertheless, it's still difficult for me to accept that Amy, in my absence, without my asking her to, cleans the shack, washes the dishes and our clothes, while living with her family within our four walls. It's good, however, because our things are safe and we can share our "riches" somewhat. Since Christian has a few Filipino friends from the middle class, we can make an excursion out of town now and again.

Our slum house, particularly the lower part made of cement, is pleasantly cool right about now. Christmas is around the corner! Everything is decorated. Colored lights give even the slum shacks and little alleys a festive air. We wish you a happy Christmas season!

Affectionate Greetings, Christine

December 21, 1994. *Dear Ones, for some time now it is very peaceful in NIA. Yesterday we bought Swiss Toblerone to give to the neighbors for Christmas. On the 24th of December we will be here in the slum. The people will go from house to house, everywhere there will be something to eat, a true community feast. Of course, there are also families who are so poor that they can't prepare anything and therefore close up their shack. On the 25th and 26th of December we will celebrate a family Christmas in the Servants house, with an artificial Christmas tree and gifts. On the 26th we will all take a trip together to a swimming pool . . . for Christmas! Over New Year's in Manila it is extremely loud and also dangerous; consequently, we're planning a few days of vacation at the beach.*

Two weeks ago we were in Mindoro, an island south of Manila, over the weekend. Recently there was a strong earthquake there. The dreamlike palm beach was not affected by the quake, but otherwise many people on the island were killed or lost their homes. In the few months that we've been in the Philippines there has been a typhoon, an earthquake, and a serious boat accident! Actually we wanted to help with an aid effort on the island, but the whole thing was canceled because the local politicians misused the help for their own propaganda.

In Mindoro I actually snorkeled for the first time. There are incredibly beautiful corals and fish here! Christian went out to sea with the fishermen in the evening. Isabel thoroughly enjoyed the shells, pieces of coral, and the sand.

Last week I visited a family from Holland in their house in the wealthy quarter. For the last three years, the young mother, Tina, has been teaching people from the villages and impoverished areas about health precaution and care. She asked me to come by now and then because Tim, her small son, has absolutely no playmates.

He is cared for all day long by a Philippine nanny. Isabel was enraptured: A giant house, many, many toys, like in paradise! Only the concept of playing together doesn't work quite yet. When Isabel has managed to get her hands on something, it doesn't occur to her to give it back to the other child. Looking around the house, I found it surprising that it is possible to lead a lifestyle here just as at home, almost without any difference. Food, décor, clothes, simply everything!

The work situations of my friends in the slum keep me busy. Most of the neighbors who have a job work seven days a week, between ten and twelve hours per day. Some sit in traffic for an additional three or four hours per day. Many employees don't have enough to do, but have to be present nonetheless. They earn about 7 Swiss francs (5 US dollars) per day or less. I had a short chat with one of the security guards, who guard shops, restaurants, banks, or other buildings. He stands from 8:00 a.m. until 8:00 p.m. in a warm uniform at the entrance of a photo shop and opens the door for the customers, with a half hour midday break. I try to imagine how slowly the time must pass in this kind of work. . . .

Love, your Christine

At Home in NIA

Now it is March. From May on, temperatures over 100 degrees will prevail here. In our little chamber on the ground floor, a fluorescent light is on continuously. Daylight has been obstructed by add-on construction to accommodate the increasing number of new arrivals in the lower regions of the slums where we are living. In return, it is distinctly cooler down here than in the incubator above, under the tin roof.

Whatever we want to begin here, we are to make happen together with the Filipinos. We have the contacts. Jesse and Lenny, who live in the Frisco slum, and Pastor Noel Gabaldon, a slim, charismatic bachelor, who lives on a wooden bench in his little chapel and stores all of his belongings in a cardboard box under the bench. In addition, Pastor Pepe and his wife, Baby, from Navotas. And, of course, Joshua Palma, a theology student and lay pastor of a Baptist community, who lives on Smokey Mountain and in NIA. He has become a true friend.

It is always a great pleasure when old acquaintances from the congregations and projects in Potrero or Bagong Silang visit us. Often they have expectations of me, but as sorry as I am, I have to hold myself apart from what is happening in those areas. Others have taken on the responsibilities there, and with Christine and Isabel in my life, a new chapter has begun. Despite that, old friendships naturally endure.

A regular visitor is Jojie Cesista, the hero of Potrero, who saved his lazy nephew from "lynch justice." He has married in the meantime, has two children, and lives in the countryside near the city. Twice already, he has brought us fresh fish, although his family hardly has enough to subsist. His tuberculosis has returned with a vengeance; even his daughter now has the disease. I plan to ask friends in Switzerland to take on the expenses of their treatment. It's good that he doesn't live in NIA; no one knows him here, and therefore no jealousy will fester.

We took a short trip not long ago with my former bodyguards, who lived in the "Orphanage" five years ago: Dario, Noriel, Reymond, and Brian. Most of them now have a family, and a few are faithful coworkers in the Bagong Silang Community. Almost all work hard to try to earn their living. Their daily wages are hardly enough to satisfy their basic needs. That makes me feel wretched.

Letter from Manila

April 4, 1995. My Dear Ones, in the shack across the way (eight feet away), a violent fight is raging. I always think of the children who are beaten in the fury. The parents are overwhelmed by their situation, drink too much or take drugs in order to forget the daily misery. That makes everything even worse, and I have to listen and can't help. How depressing!

Last week I gave a woman milk and some money, knowing that her child, the same age as Isabel, was sick and hungry. Later she told me that on that very evening she cried out to God in despair because she simply had no pesos in her purse.

Kind regards, Christine

The Mountain of Rubbish

I still feel as if I'm in shock. A couple of men from NIA work in refuse collection and every morning bring their full trucks to a somewhat distant, open dump site at the edge of our area of the city. According to government statistics, the adjacent slum, Payatas, has 300,000 residents. Yesterday, I was allowed to go with them in a garbage truck: A short hour later and we were at the highest point of a sixty-five to one-hundred feet high and a half-mile long rubbish mountain.

There I stood in the middle of hundreds of people who, with special steel hooks and with bare hands under the brooding heat of the sun, searched for valuables buried in the city's rubbish—a silent performance within a noisy scene of bellowing diesel motors belonging to dredgers and trucks that thundered onto the scene in syncopated rhythm, and deposited tons of disgusting, stinking garbage onto the mountain. There were children and old people among the garbage pickers, some wrapped in rags, with bent backs and inflamed eyes, and wounds or sores covered with flies. A few had bandaged their faces with rags and were masked, to protect themselves from the dust in the air and from the pitiless sun, and perhaps also in shame, from the glances of the curious. It is beyond difficult to describe.

Some days later I speak to Joshua, in Tondo, where the well-known garbage dump site known as Smokey Mountain is located. Joshua is the "thinker" of the neighborhood organization Akbayan, which represents about 2,000 families of scavengers.

"Smokey Mountain was a constant eyesore of the Aquino and Ramos governments," Joshua tells me. In 1991, it was planned to transform the land into an expensive industrial and shopping zone and to construct blocks of public housing for the residents. But the majority resisted, and their non-violent resistance was reported worldwide throughout the media. The response of the mighty soon became obvious. On May 8, 1992 a fire of 'unknown origin' destroyed half of the slum shacks. A couple of weeks later, our spokesman was shot to death."

I ask Joshua why the scavengers continue to maintain their undignified lives.

"Mainly *because* of their feelings of self-worth," Joshua says. "We don't want to be at anyone's mercy or to fall short. We have the desire for a piece of land from which we will not be driven away. If we had a choice, the mountain of rubbish would never have become our lasting pursuit. But in our provinces, the government did not start any development programs; our fathers were left to their fate. So now we are here. And you know what? We scavengers had no voice in the planning of our future. To this day, we have no written promise that we will actually receive assistance from the settlement program that has been announced. We recognize the empty promises of the government."

Letter from Manila

May 23, 1995. *My Dear Ones, for approximately two months we have been reading the Bible on Sunday evening with two or three neighbors. My language aide and new friend Jessica participates. On Wednesday evening we meet for prayers and discussion with Jesse and Lenny Sarol, Joshua and soon, we hope, with other Filipinos. We would like to live and work more closely with the Filipinos.*

In our little house we again have large rats, especially at night. They leave droppings behind, in addition to all of the other dirt that we have to deal with: soot, dust, dog excrement in front of the shack, urine on the wall of every house. . . . Christian has no choice but to set traps again and to drown the rats, which he doesn't like to do.

Also sapping our strength are the many visitors that often rain down upon us around noon, keeping us from the urgently necessary midday nap. Despite everything, it's great that we can maintain so many contacts without traveling far. Many visitors undertake the three to four hour trip from Bagong Silang, without knowing if we will be at home. When we are away, the neighbors let them come into our shack. . . .

Kind regards, Christine

Culture Shock

Eight months have passed since our arrival. For some days now, Christine has been suffering from a kind of culture shock. It is a mixture of weariness, depression, and a desire to flee into another reality, because everything is a little too much for her. I had a similar experience that time in Bagong Silang . . . with the difference that I wasn't pregnant then, in contrast to Christine today!

Just as one would expect, now in July, when it's still very hot but the rain season has begun, our fluorescent light is dark and our fan isn't moving. They're saying that a transformer exploded. In the night I saw that the steel canisters at the cable junctions were glowing red because too many people were illegally poaching the electrical current. A kind of slum syndicate has "organized" the conduits, and the poor pay them—most certainly more than the rich outside the slums. Now a money collector will soon come by to drum up additional *pesos* for a new transformer. Until then, our clothes will stick to our bodies.

I try, overall, to remain positive, and to relieve Christine wherever necessary and possible. Naturally, I am fascinated by the evaluation of various potential projects; the dream of better times is a helpful diversion in these times of seemingly endless desert. Fortunately, Isabel is fine. She has become a delightful little chatterbox, but despite our efforts, speaks hardly a word of German, only pure Tagalog.

Three weeks ago I introduced Joshua and his people to our attorneys that work with Harry Roque. On the Sunday before last, Harry took a couple of representatives of Akbayan to his congregation's service and introduced him to the rector, who is not only Harry's friend but also the spiritual advisor of President Ramos. They gave the rector a letter to be delivered to the President.

In October, we will be here a year, and our introductory year into the language and culture will end. Yes, we feel at home here in our slum neighborhood. I'm already thinking about how our Filipino friends and we can help the boys from the streets in a deliberate, targeted way. Working with young people or providing life lessons are costly. We must try to build our own financial sources, perhaps with the purchase of a large air conditioned bus for group transport as an income generating project.

The Payatas Gang

Last week Jesse, Lenny, and I watched "While You Were Sleeping" with Sandra Bullock in the movie theater of the pleasantly cool shopping mall. Nice entertainment, without blood and violence and almost without tears; the director of the film is not named Jon Turteltaub [Turtledove] for nothing. In the night we heard shots near our shack. And in the chapel once again lies the corpse of a young man who officially has died of fish poisoning, but actually by the "lynch justice" of the police. Bad fish does not cause wounds in the head . . . How perverse the world is here: For murder and manslaughter in Switzerland one has to go to the movies. Here one has to leave the movie theater.

The Payatas mountain of rubbish occupies my time. I have put together some numbers regarding the slum near this pile of rubble that make me quite unhappy: Some 300,000 people live on 740 acres there; 47 percent of them are unemployed.

The rate of population growth lies at 15 percent. Some 50 percent of children are poorly or under-nourished, 80 percent of the inhabitants do not own their own toilet. Many more than 1,000 families live here, directly on the slope of the dump site, on which they gather and sort trash, and sell for reuse. And: More than 1,000 tons of trash is unloaded here—daily!

A few weeks ago I made contact with several "jumpers." They are eight- to twelve-year-old boys who jump on and off the trucks, tossing the rubbish back and forth, sorting items of potential value for the driver before the garbage reaches the trash heap. The jumpers left school long ago and are glue sniffers. Their work is dirty and dangerous, but they love their liberty, bought with the few *pesos* that they earn for themselves. A number of them are dressed only in rags and clearly undernourished.

I've brought them sandwiches and fruit juice a few times at the access road where the boys wait for the trucks. And now, my friend Lito from NIA and Franklin, the brother of Jesse, and I planned an excursion for the jumpers to a river and reservoir about forty-five minutes away from the dump. As we arrived at the appointed time at the usual street corner, with a guitar and a super picnic, not a single jumper was to be seen far and wide. I was disappointed. Perhaps they thought that the swimming outing was a ruse and we would put them in a home instead; or, that we were resistance fighters who round up children and force them to become soldiers. Or pedophiles, or child traffickers. Such experiences are also a part of the lives of these forgotten children!

We waited for an hour and then gave up. After a prayer for the children and a prayer to God for clarity about what we would do next, we drove undecided along the edge of the slum. Then, at a corner, we noticed a group of youths in an exuberant mood.

We approached them: "Do you have any interest in coming with us to go swimming? We have friends that . . . uh . . . have been prevented from coming, and we have some room." This was not particularly original (even somewhat "pedophile") in approach. Nonetheless, rather than being mistrusting, the boys hollered and hooted. Suddenly, it became clear to me that most of them were drunk or drugged. But there was no going back; they were already tearing open the doors to our small bus and storming inside.

"Yikes," shot through my brain, "this was probably not the answer to our prayer. . . ."

And so we sat in the delivery van, Lito and Franklin and I, together with a group of sixteen- to nineteen-year-old wild types, who were celebrating a birthday with beer and liquor. Franklin played the guitar, everyone sang and caroused and drummed rhythmically on the body of the bus. The atmosphere in the car was super.

Arriving at the river, they jumped into the cool and cloudy water in their underwear and in high spirits, playing like little children. Then we sat in the sand and devoured the sandwiches and cake with fruit juice. Now they wanted to know who we actually were. We were Christians and wanted to help young people on the slope of the rubbish mountain, we said, even though we didn't quite know how.

The reactions of the boys was astounding. They began to tell us about their lives. They all were scavengers and part of a gang. Their boss and spokesman was John, a dark wiry type, with a handsome, masculine face. Only a couple of them ever attended school, and that was years ago. Their families had thrown them out, they said, because they only caused trouble.

As we later said goodbye near the shacks at the rubbish heap, we had to promise that we would come again. And suddenly I knew that this encounter was no coincidence. God had master minded a great little story here.

Rain Season

It has been raining without interruption for the last few weeks. Our shack smells moldy, like an unventilated cellar. We are slowly getting used to it. In return, the stink of the wastewater in the open at our front door isn't as penetrating because it's diluted by the rain. This evening, gloomy thoughts pervade the atmosphere. On October 28, the day before yesterday, they violently removed the slum settlement on Smokey Mountain. Some days before, Nestor, the spokesman and vice president of Akbayan, asked the appropriate authorities for a reprieve, whereupon the representative of the government promised to delay permission for any demolition until after further public negotiations with Akbayan.

But then, the day before yesterday, some 3,000 men appeared—police and enforcement troops in civilian dress. In anticipation, the scavengers had wisely erected barricades. Despite the barricade, Nestor said that if the police produced a demolition order, he would compel the residents to leave the settlement without resistance. "Order from the top, without paper," the police responded and began to tear down the barricades. Joshua says that the violent clash was terrible. On the side of the garbage pickers there were two fatalities, among them a small child, and nineteen wounded. According to the newspaper, on the side of the police there were a couple of lacerations and abrasions.

Something else also troubles me: Our relationship with Servants. The idea to buy an air conditioned bus has not been well received by the Servants team:

The project is too big, they say; it's moving too quickly. For us, the regular interaction with these colleagues is very important; they are a part of our own Servants identity. In the last weeks we have had numerous discussions with the team leadership in which we were deliberately transparent. During this time, it became ever clearer to us that with our vision and our resolute advancement, we would no longer have a place on the Servants team in Manila.

Now the team leadership has advised us that our probationary period should be extended, so that we would have another opportunity to align our ideas with the Servants' philosophy.

At this moment, it's raining not only outside; it's also raining in me.

Doubly Pregnant

Christine is getting rounder and rounder, and not because of the Christmas feast two weeks ago!

The Christmas season in 1995 was noisy and cheerful, but somewhat overshadowed. Isabel suffered with dengue, a critical viral illness with a high fever and danger of hemorrhaging. And the previous violent evacuation of Joshua and his scavengers had seriously eclipsed the festive atmosphere. Nonetheless, we look toward the next year full of expectations. Not only is Christine pregnant, but so am I—thanks to Christine's parents!

We enjoyed a few days with them at the sea in the well-known tourist resort of Puerto Galera. Remote sandy beaches, rainforest with waterfalls, fresh air. I had to think again and again of our friends in the slums. How *they* would enjoy and relax in this place, the street children and young people, if they for once could see the sky without the gray veil of the big city's soot! I could see them in front of me, running into the clear ocean waters with the colorful fish; I could hear them shouting in delight. They would learn to know creation and also its Creator from a completely new vantage point.

As we strolled along the beach with Christine's parents one morning, I pointed to a large house made of bamboo with a giant straw roof. It stands on a particularly idyllic site, built on solid cliffs and fits nicely under the palms.

"That is the Spaghetti House," I said, "a tourist magnet belonging to a Swiss man. It's for sale. One should have such a house—then one could invite the poor from Manila."

"Why don't you buy it?" my parents-in-law asked. "We'll lend you the money!"

I could feel how the blood raced to my head. It is not their style to make such jokes. And I had only fantasized aloud. I had never considered my in-laws to be people who had much extra money. But they were serious.

In the meantime Christine's parents are back in Switzerland. But their words continue to have resonance. If that was an offer from God, then it came just at the right time.

The tensions with the leadership of Servants had not abated, quite to the contrary. The "extended probationary period" made clear how different our visions are. On that side, the foreign Servants, on this side, our Filipino friends and we. For them, we are too impatient. For us, their guiding principles are too narrow and rigid. We, with our desire for action and our willingness to take risks, constantly run into resistance, and it will most likely remain that way.

I don't really know where their problem with us actually lies. From our perspective, we follow the five principles of Servants in our lives: Incarnation (living with the poor), Simplicity (modest lifestyle), Community (to live and work together), Servanthood (to serve and empower), Wholism (to live and preach grace and justice). I think they could certainly afford us some elbow room and implicit trust.

In the last weeks we visited the rubbish slope in Payatas regularly. We now have a deeper relationship with the adolescent gang. That gives us power.

Letter from Manila

February 13, 1996. *To give birth without full anesthesia and caesarean section is very unusual here—except for the poor. We had to participate, therefore, in a special course in "Lamaze"—the breathing technique—with a final exam! When I entered the clinic the doctors asked me with great concern if I really dared to give birth to my child without anesthesia. My female gynecologist thought she would never be able to do it—at the least, she would need an epidural anesthetic! I believe Filipinas are somewhat more sensitive to pain than European women. But, it really does hurt.*

The pains set in during a meeting on Saturday afternoon. I left the meeting at the break, strolled home, baked a loaf of bread as provision for Chris and entertained a group of the neighbors' children who wanted to play at our place. After we dropped Isabel at Amy's, Chris and I drove to the Servants house at five o'clock in the evening. There the pains began to come every six to seven minutes, but not so strong that I felt we had to leave for the hospital immediately. Chris became nervous, however, so we packed the little suitcase and made our way there. Christian Auer drove us, and we had barely arrived when everything started.

On Sunday morning at 5:22 a.m., Noel was here. They took us to a private room with a second bed for relations who would take care of the patient. Noel remained at the newborn's station for about six hours before I could have him in the room. There after Noel's care by the hospital was concluded, other than taking his temperature and checking on his weight a couple of times.

Actually the birth and also the three-day "childbed" were a better experience than that in Switzerland. During the birth the same doctors were always present; there are no midwives in the hospital. Altogether I had three or four people around me and of course, Chris. Also the care provided to patients by next-of-kin—in my case, Chris, and from time to time our Servants housemother Rita Ringma—was very comforting.

In addition we stayed in the Servants house for three days. How nice that I always had someone to chat with there, different than in Basel, where I was all alone in the apartment. Here in NIA it's like that too. I feel generally happy and already really physically fit!

Kind regards, Christine

The Vision "Onesimo"

February 20, 1996. We don't belong to Servants Manila any longer. All the discussions, in which I had hoped that *both sides* could draw nearer to one another in the laying out of their principles, broke down.

Despite pain and disappointment we are happy that for the most part, we could resolve the conflict objectively. The leadership of Servants offered us the opportunity to take part in the regular fellowship meetings with the team in the future. We gratefully accepted! At least we won't lose our ongoing friendships with the remaining coworkers.

In the meantime we are engaged in founding a Philippine foundation acknowledged as a private charity engaged in voluntary social work. At a prayer retreat with our Philippine coworkers Jesse and Lenny, Joshua, Pepe and Baby, Franklin and Noel Gabaldon, the name "Onesimo" came up, the Philippine version of the Greek name Onesimus. St. Paul writes in his short Epistle to Philemon about a slave with this name who as a youth was torn from his home and landed in a prison, where his life was fundamentally changed by his fellow prisoner, St. Paul.

It's exactly that which we want to do: Offer true friendship and comprehensive training to the point of eye level to young runaways, dropouts, and the abandoned or discarded, through which their life can be fundamentally changed. Together with the available network of communities of various denominations, we want to bring to life a wholly Christ-centered youth effort and leadership-training program. We want to encourage the founding of small businesses and thereby the self-help aspect of the fight against poverty. Everything should fit into the Philippine context and from the beginning be led by Filipinos. It should be done under the umbrella of a foundation. And the foundation is to be called Onesimo.

Make Way for Camp Rock

Fundamental change is brewing! We were at the beach over the weekend with our Philippine friends and spoke with them about our vision—to buy the Spaghetti House in order to offer youth leisure activities, leadership courses, and weeks of training seminars. We deliberated, discussed, and prayed. Finally all decided to carry the project forward together. Now we have named the house and the 8,600 square feet of surrounding land "Camp Rock." Our faithful friend and attorney Harry Roque will wind up the purchase. The seller has allowed us to use the grounds immediately. I feel a tingling. . . .

Another tingling is also under way: At the beginning of May we will move to the Frisco slum into the lower floor of a solidly built cement brick shack. We have two small rooms there, not far from Jesse and Lenny Sarol and almost

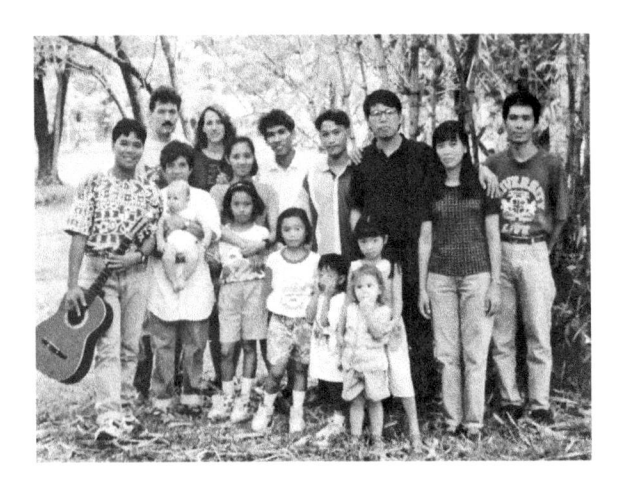

The beginnings of Onesimo. From left to right: Jesse, Christian, Lenny, Christine, Olen and Noel, Willi, Pepe and Baby, Joshua.

next to the chapel of Pastor Noel Gabaldon. The closeness that we seek is finally palpable.

Frisco is somewhat larger than NIA; there are about two- to three-thousand families in residence there. The slum lies on a river, the only giant wastewater canal, which in the rain season regularly floods everything in the surrounding area. On the land side, a fifteen-foot high fireproof wall delineates the slum—a half circle—from the area of a paint factory. A single access street serves the approximately ten- to fifteen-thousand people. We live in the back part of the slum in a kind of a dead-end alley. If there were to be a fire in the slum and panic ensue, we would probably have to jump into the river.

Our domicile is a little more difficult to access and the surroundings seem a little less friendly than NIA, but instead we have more space and no wastewater directly in front of the door—at least in the dry season.

Our conflict with the leadership of the Servants in Manila engendered several clarifying discussions, that is, exchange of written correspondence, with the organization Servants Switzerland. Fortunately, our Swiss friends trust us going forward and also wish to provide support to our foundation, Onesimo. The founding is well under way, and we are in contact with professionals and intellectuals of the Philippine middle-class who are being considered for the governing body of the foundation.

This evening I will compose a circulating letter for our Swiss friends to inform them about the state of affairs here. I will ask them for 75,000 franks as starting capital for our projected transport undertaking. And then we will plan the first leisure activities for young people at Camp Rock.

"Your Shack is on Fire!"

Tuesday, April 16, 1996. In the evening at half past eight, we sit post event, discussing our first leisure activities program at Camp Rock. We are happy that we may use the Servants house now as before. A good mood prevails on all sides.

The first organization of leisure time, a kind of exercise with seven of our wild boys from Payatas was an experience. Alehandro had, for the first time in his seventeen years of life, left the slum, seen clear water in the rainforest, a beach without garbage, a sun without a veil of foul gasses, a new world. All of the boys learned something about the love of Jesus of Nazareth during this week.

Intensive preparations for the actual leisure time activities took place. A two-day leadership school, in which approximately thirty teenagers entrusted themselves to one another and to God, was the high point. Approximately 200 youths from eight poverty-stricken areas took part in the activities phase with the theme "Young People, Awaken!" The girls slept in the house, the boys built themselves a little tent village on the beach. We experimented with program elements that our Filipino friends did not know, such as a job track with the theme of gifts and talents, and a night track of group devotional exercises. The adventure program according to a biblical theme was a real high point.

In the midst of this joyful post discussion of the week's activities, the telephone rang: "There's a fire in NIA, come quickly, your shack, too, is quickly burning to the ground! We don't know exactly where Isabel is." My heart begins to race. Isabel is with Amy and Benjie in the best care, but if our shack is burning, so is theirs.

After a break-neck drive I stumble through the smoking wreckage of NIA, forcing myself along soot-smeared faces. "Stay calm, whatever you come across," I pant at myself. Then I bump into Benjie, and . . . Oh, miraculously, our as-built intertwined shacks are empty and flooded with extinguishing water but intact. The fire turned away just a few feet in front of our huts and moved in another direction—just as in a cheap Hollywood film, only real! Isabel is unhurt. Benjie first brought the children to safety and then threw his and our belongings over the adjacent wall.

The next morning the measure of the calamity became clearer: Between 500 and 800 families have lost everything. A picture to make one weep and despair—without electricity or water and with the many homeless in NIA everything is upside down. And Christine is in the last stages of recovering from the flu. We determine to stay at Servants house until our move to Frisco.

Naturally we take part in the coordination of quick response. The slum lacks everything—nutritional products, clothing, dishes, building material for new roofs. At this time of year, the sun burns especially without pity. The people are enormously brave. Marked by lack of sleep and despair, they carry building debris out to the street, or confused, dig around in the ashes. I fax a short report to our communities in Switzerland.

The government organizes nourishment for the first five days. I search in vain for a report in the daily newspaper about the fire. As if fires in the slum were part of daily life! Many are convinced that the government started the fire, since such misfortune hastens the planned dispersal of the poor to the outskirts of the city.

On Sunday we sit in the little chapel in NIA, which was also saved from the fire. "God is good, God is good, God is so good, so good to me . . . ," the people sing. The hymn seems to pass their lips sincerely, while I sit and doubt God's goodness. Tearful reports of preservation and mourning follow. At a minimum, ten families of the congregation have lost all their belongings. A man explains to me in a shaky voice, "Now I understand what Jesus meant when he said we should not gather treasures on earth, but rather in heaven."

On Wednesday, a phone call from Switzerland reaches me. Upon our fax, the congregation of our church has spontaneously collected money and has "plundered" the community cash box and will send us 18,000 francs (14,580 US dollars) as immediate help. Together with other donations and the Servants Project money at hand, we can provide 38,000 francs (30,780 US dollars) as immediate help without delay. Unbelievable!

We organize a discussion with communal prayers, as to how we can best use this money without provoking jealousy. Pastor B. G. Polidario from the small Christian community in NIA produces a list of the families who have suffered the greatest losses. They need, above all, a roof over their heads. The poorest are to be provided with building materials.

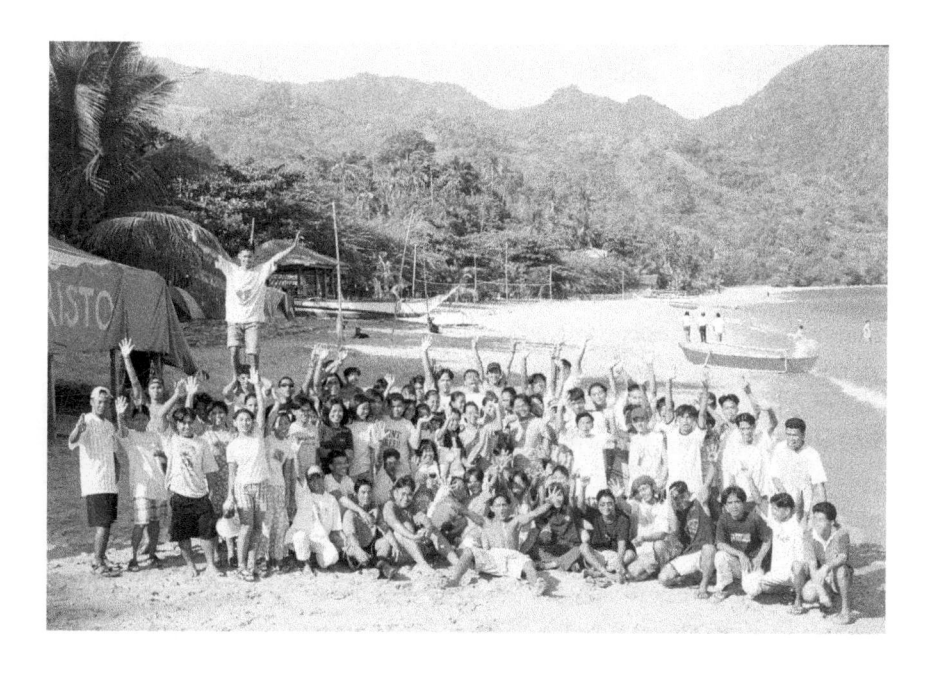

At the first Leisure Program with the theme, "Kabatann Gising!" (Young People, Awake!) approximately 200 young people from eight impoverished areas took part.

Noteworthy Contrasts

Yesterday, May 26, 1996, we officially founded the Onesimo Foundation Incorporated and had it registered as a non-governmental organization in the Philippines. Visions and goals of the organization are formulated. The director is Noel Gabaldon, the pastor, who lives in his chapel diagonally across the street from our little house in the Frisco slum. The president of the Foundation is our lawyer Harry Roque; active in the leadership in addition to us is a social worker, a doctor and psychiatrist, a dentist, a pastor and a psychologist.

Our new residence in Frisco will soon be a series of changing feelings—high-low, up-down. For example, there are our neighbors. They're pleasant, certainly, but for the most part people who have sunk deeply into the vicious circle of poverty, disease, and violence. The "owner" of our slum house who lives in the upper story directly above us, was friendly and forthcoming right from the beginning. Of course, he is *the* drug dealer in all of Frisco—which of course we've only now found out. Recently his wife, Ate Gilda, asked us for an advance payment of our rent which she needed to get her husband out of prison—he had been arrested. Since we want to stay in Frisco a minimum of one year, we paid her the year's rent. The man has been free again for the last few days, and in the meantime we found out why they took him into custody: He was procuring clients for an underage prostitute, whose father reported him to the police. Our landlord is also a pimp.

Ate Gilda comes downstairs to see us when she's in distress. We listen patiently to her crazy worries and pray with her, since that is her express wish. Her life hardly appears to change because of it. We have noticed that she is obviously addicted to crystal meth. While we here below read the Bible and sing, above us something that can only be described as a drug and sex party is going on. This juxtaposition is one of many noteworthy aspects of our daily existence.

Our little Noel couldn't be better! He is an undemanding, blue-eyed little boy, who bestows an enchanting smile on his surroundings. On Sunday before last, we had him blessed in the Philippine tradition, with a festive little neighborhood get-together.

Noel is not the only addition to our family: Ron, a fifteen-year-old from the rubbish mountain has moved in with us. He was so undernourished that he could hardly stand up. Since he's gotten a bit better, he has shown a happy and helpful temperament and is attached to us like an eight-year-old pulled from the floods. His emotional level is several years behind his actual age. At the same time, Jessica, Christine's eighteen-year-old language aide, who moved from NIA to Frisco, is also living with us. Now we speak Tagalog in the house more often.

We recently became aware how tired we are. The conflict regarding our disengagement from Servants in Manila has drained us emotionally more than we would care to admit. Onesimo, the big youth camp, the quick move from NIA, the fire, the purchase of Camp Rock, which became quite protracted—it's all a little too much at the same time.

Much more pleasant are encounters such as one recently with Ate Juliet, the head of the kindergarten in the stilts house and cemetery slum in Navotas. I visited her because I had heard that the school had been excluded from the alliance of Christian preschools founded by the Servants.

The slum with its smell of decay is very unpleasant, the graves with their boxes of the dead intermingled with the brittle plywood shacks of the living; heavy trucks unload their trash into the sea illegally, and therefore mostly at night. But the courageous Ate Juliet doesn't let it affect her, and keeps the school running in full operation: "After the exclusion from the alliance I let the parents know that the school would be closed. Suddenly they awakened, paid their tuition and became actively involved. Now so many children come that I have to teach a class each morning and afternoon."

What a story: The poorest school, which was excluded from the alliance, had developed into the only really independent "Learning Center." I am really proud of Juliet and her crew. I promise her that we would provide the metal door that she needs to keep vandals at bay.

Sometimes Heaven Helps . . .

It has been five months since the fire in NIA. Pastor B. G. and his team of locals were actually able to convert the donations from Europe into genuine aid without arousing jealousy or incurring any losses. Some 800 families received immediate help in the form of food and the most necessary household goods. An additional 430 families received corrugated tin, plywood planks, and similar building materials. The small chapel was able to be expanded with an addition of a larger room for a kindergarten. Finally, NIA's neighborhood association also received some building material for a small guardhouse.

On the other hand, the situation at Smokey Mountain does not look as good. A majority of the residents is living in the provisional shelters provided by the government for its use; a minority, however, is occupying a few blocks of vacant houses. Every day, approximately 300 members of Akbayan sit and protest in front of the grand Cathedral of the City of Manila and hold open-air worship services with banners and processions. They demand recompense from the government for the victims of the violent resettlement of October 28, 1995; support in search of a living wage for those formerly active as scavengers; free lodging in public housing or at the least, affordable rent, which would then be applied to development projects.

Nestor, the vice president and deacon of the community, is living in hiding. He is accused of having shot a man who died during the resettlement-by-force with the intention of pinning the guilt on the police. How absurd! Now he is hopeful that with the termination of the investigation, the warrant for his arrest will be lifted.

The protest in front of the cathedral actually turns out to be successful. The media finally report on the subject of poverty in the metropolis and even place themselves ever more clearly on the side of the Smokey Mountain residents. Two members of congress as well as several organizations of the "urban poor" now actively support the demands of Akbayan. Experienced human rights attorneys offer their help free of charge! Why is it that nothing happens until the pressure of the media is brought to bear?

Some of the former residents of the Smokey Mountain settlement have reported their experience of God's presence during the evacuation battle. The brother of the pastor of the Baptist community told of a bullet that had pierced his thigh. The police continued to beat him, but suddenly he clearly felt a strange force, as if someone were carrying him, so that he could run away despite the bullet. If one were to read something like that in the newspaper, one would dismiss it as a fantastic story. But when the person in question himself tells the story, his eyes welling with tears of gratitude, only a callous cynic would not believe him.

I am so grateful for the air conditioned bus that we bought and renovated during the summer, and "consecrated" with the boys from the slums. A short time ago, we set it up as a public conveyance. It provided five jobs, two for our coworkers, and soon it is to carry the ongoing expenses of Onesimo. In order to avoid unnecessary risks, we intend to build our little transportation business slowly and carefully. Because of corruption at all levels, and because of the often questionable work ethic, honest businesses are very difficult to maintain.

The financing of the bus is an answered prayer. The money was gathered together within a few weeks. Many small contributions were collected, and beyond belief, also a gigantic donation—30,000 francs (24,300 US dollars)—from an acquaintance living in Switzerland. She wrote us that her car had caught fire on the highway and was totally demolished, but she herself survived the accident without harm. With the incident still uppermost in her thoughts, she sat down in a nearby church, thanked God, and considered the fact that she was about to spend 30,000 francs on a new car. Then our solicitation Letter to Friends came to mind, and she decided that our bus was more important than her car. What largesse! Heaven seems to find ways to support our work. We feel validated in our bus project.

Naturally there are also small every-day disillusionments. The experience of the wonderful first leisure-activity program at Camp Rock a few months ago was less enduring than I anticipated. A few of the boys from Payatas, for example, actually did get an idea as to who God is and how much he loves them. They returned with the firm resolution to begin a new life. However, their usual daily activities in the slum and on the streets quickly drew them in again—failed relationships, glue sniffing, crystal meth, alcohol. I believe that above all, I underestimated the severe drug addiction of the boys.

It can't be done with terrific camps alone. We would have to have them under our intensive care for much longer periods. We would have to develop a systematic guidance program, a training school for life, a kind of therapeutic communal living arrangement with clear goals. We would have to undertake a "journey" together. For that we would need a house and a competent team. And, of course, God.

. . . and Sometimes a Revolver

The purchase of Camp Rock proceeds slowly. Nevertheless, the authorities finally measured the land a few days ago. How we reached that point is a story unto itself.

Three weeks ago I climb into the bus at 4:00 a.m. in Quezon City for a two-day excursion to Camp Rock. I want to arrange for permits from the local government on the island of Mindoro for a number of improvements to begin to be made to the holiday house there. The driver turns on the diesel motor to summon the passengers to board.

"Do I have time to get a cup of coffee?" I ask him.

"Just," he answers.

So I charge toward the brand new donut-coffee shop, whose glowing neon light beckons me. In my haste, I don't notice that a spanking-new glass wall has been erected across the entire front of the restaurant to keep out the smut of the bus station. With full force, I slam my forehead into the glass front and fall to the floor. The fancy lady at the counter is horrified and begins to scream. I am lying in shards of glass, blood is flowing down my face and over my clothes. My right hand is split open by a deep laceration.

As I get up, I become dizzy and stumble outside. Four taxis are parked there, all with open doors, but none of the drivers wants to take me. "I'll pay extra, I have to go to the hospital . . . ," I shout. A young man comes to my aid: "I'll make a deal with one of them, don't worry. . . ."

The driver who finally takes me to the hospital has his seats covered in plastic and during the trip explains to me in dramatic terms how horrible I look and how it is a bad omen if a customer should die in the vehicle. Splendid.

I know the emergency room of St. Luke's Medical Center from various "emergencies" and from the birth of Noel. St. Luke's is among the best hospitals in the land, with deluxe suites for the super rich on the penthouse floor. A friendly young physician's assistant cleans my wounds and shaves my hair around a deep, circular cut just under the hair line. "I'll sew up the head wound myself," he says," but the wound on the hand looks more complicated. I'll call the chief physician."

At first, the chief physician seems very sleepy. While he pokes around the wound with the anesthesia needle, he begins to wake up and ask questions: How did the accident occur, where do I come from, why am I living in the Philippines, and so forth. He bends deeply over my hand and chatters happily while spraying saliva into the open wound. I carefully ask why he isn't wearing a surgical mask.

"Young man," he says, "I complain all the time about the lack of medicinal material at this station. We're supposedly the best hospital in the country—and have no surgical masks at present. It's a joke, no?" And while he sews the sinew to the thumb, he laughs cheerfully and blathers on into the wound.

At 9:00 a.m., I finally climb into the bus to Mindoro: with twelve stitches in my forehead, ten in my hand, with painkillers and a super dose of antibiotics, which will most likely deal with the chief physician's oral germs. In Switzerland, after such an accident, one would be laid up for a few days. But I don't want to return to the slum and sit around. And with head and hand bandages here in the bus, I'm not worried about more or less attention. As an Amerikano, one attracts enough as it is.

The current owner of our piece of land—Camp Rock—is Mr. Solario, a dignified older gentleman with a stern glance, prominent chin and cheek bones—an ardent gambler. The Solarios own and occupy the large tourist resort adjacent to the Camp Rock property. Most people address him as "Captain," because he was apparently the captain of a ship earlier in his life. The Solarios want to see our dollars, finally, since our camp is already set up there. In order for the purchase contract to become effective and the entry into the land register to take place, however, the property must first be officially measured. But the official assessor has, to date, conducted such a slovenly survey without taking responsibility for its completion, that the Captain, opening the passenger's door of his new Landrover, waves me inside and growls, "We're going to take this vagabond on!"

Mr. Solario is slightly tipsy, as usual, and I'm not exactly comfortable with the situation. On the other hand, the purchase of the property has to be accomplished, finally, and I'm also angry with this assessor, a powerful, corrupt, large, fat man with a macho attitude and an aura that gives one the shivers; and who makes pointed reference to the fact that one is completely dependent on his good graces and that a nice honorarium would possibly encourage him to take the survey in the near future.

We lurch over marshy water buffalo paths on private property through forests of coconut palms, reach a paved private road, and arrive at a somewhat sequestered villa on a well-cared-for beach. "Here Mr. Assessor plays tennis with his rich friends in the afternoons, instead of pursuing his work," the Captain growls. As a matter of fact, we see the sweaty assessor with his racket, chasing a ball on his private tennis court.

"One moment, Captain," he wheezes, breathlessly, as he discovers us at the edge of the court, "just this set—I'll be right there." Solario strides back and forth like a tiger in his cage. As the honorable assessor finally arrives to greet us, the captain blows his top.

"I've paid you enough and waited long enough," he shouts at the assessor. "You'll survey our property next week or I'll kill you, understand?!" Then he pulls a revolver from under his Barong shirt and brandishes it about.

"Okay, okay, Mr. Solario," the assessor tries to laugh, and dabs pearls of sweat from his forehead. "We take them in order; can't accommodate everyone at once."

The Captain doesn't say another word, puts the weapon away, and marches to the Landrover. We get in and drive away. My heart is racing almost as fast as the Landrover.

A week later: The property has been surveyed. Thanks be to God—and perhaps the revolver!

A Therapeutic Communal Organization

Our bus project is somewhat of a disappointment. I now know why we have not made a profit to date. On the night before the bus was delivered to us, quite a few valuable parts were removed and replaced with scrap. Expensive repairs followed, but we have no way of proving anything.

Later we found out that the transport police had constantly been demanding payment of penalties because the bus-line license was allegedly falsified. Naturally, the police allowed the bus to continue on its way with the knowledge that they could stop it again at any time, which of course they did regularly. In fact, the penalties were bribes; the money went to corrupt policemen rather than to Onesimo!

Harry advises that we not pursue a lawsuit against the seller of the bus: We probably would not be successful but would be engaged in a long process with high costs. The team is searching intensely for a valid long-distance license or for private transport contracts with schools or business firms. My friend who is in charge of the project believes that this would be possible. But now, because of a crack in the engine block, the motor is disabled and we have to buy a substitute motor. Altogether, the total expense amounts to about 50,000 francs (40,500 US dollars). I am glad that we used only the donations explicitly intended for the bus; we had informed our contributors about the risk inherent in this undertaking.

My friends reassure me that every business transaction has its difficulties. Although the venture has not produced any profit, it did provide six employment opportunities that support a number of families. The project supervisor is the most competent of my Filipino friends by far and will no doubt sort this all out.

But there is also good news: Our concept for a therapeutic communal organization is taking form—excellent form! We are in the process of transforming a derelict shack into a habitable slum house, which will cost approximately 4,000 francs (3,240 US dollars). This Onesimo house is only a few steps away from our own lodgings. The original owners, the Formilleza family with their gifted daughter, Hazel, will take the upper story; the ground floor will have plenty of space for the communal organization. The guiding team includes: Pastor Noel Gabaldon; Franklyn Sarol, a recent arrival from the mountain province of Banawe; Willi and Rolly, two teenagers from Frisco who have been guided by Pastor Noel for two years now; William Ducos, a trusted leisure-program group-leader from the dump site of Payatas. All of them are Filipino bachelors who come from broken families, but who have already experienced a degree of healing.

We call our experiment ODT: Onesimo Discipleship Training, a six-month long life-training school for boys. It is to begin with a few days together at Camp Rock on Mindoro—to bind friendships and to withdraw from drugs. We name it "Workcamp," so that a false idea of a "beach vacation" doesn't take hold in their minds. The boys must earn their participation; they must work every morning on the building and upkeep of Camp Rock. Workcamp will be the proving ground to determine which of the twenty-five boys will be allowed to join the life-training program.

We have planned the following: In the beginning there is an official welcome. Then we provide a box where the participants can deposit their "stuff," cigarettes, knives, and other weapons, either openly or anonymously. Anyone caught with drugs or weapons, or who breaks any other rules thereafter, will be taken to the ship to Manila without warning. Otherwise it won't work.

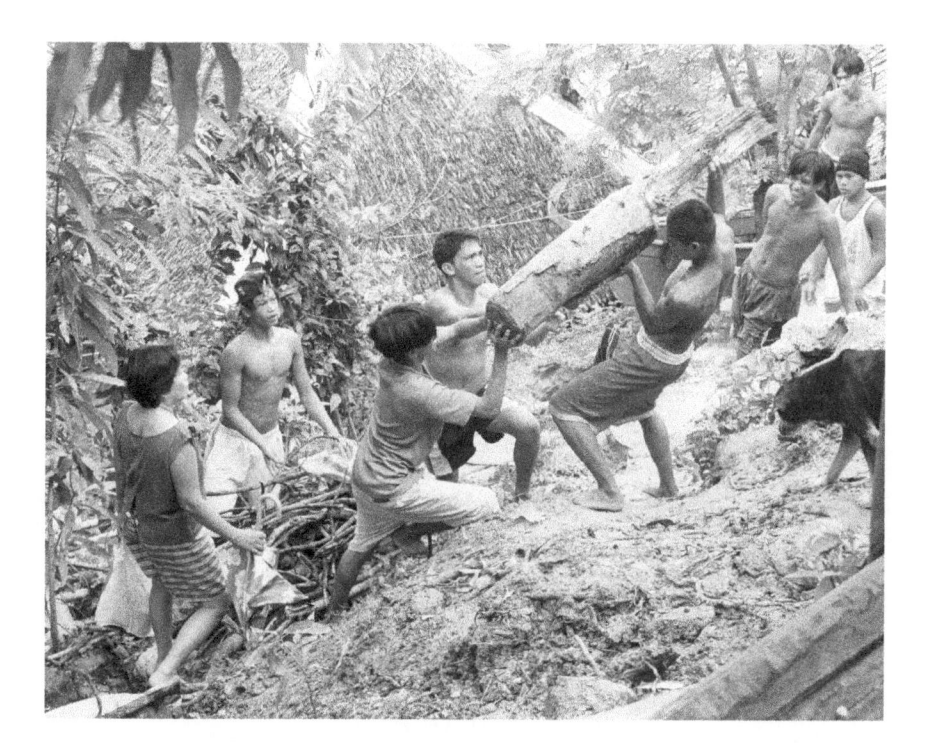

The boys must earn their participation; they work each morning on the maintenance and expansion of Camp Rock. Concurrently, it becomes clear which ones are eligible to be admitted to the residential community.

The other rules are no less clear: Everyone remains within sight on the property; no one ventures beyond. Every morning after breakfast the work in the house and on the land will be completed. In the afternoon, the program includes games, fun, swimming, basketball, mountain climbing, or sleeping. An all-you-can-eat meal is served in-between. In the evening, everyone meets to sing, discuss, and pray. Participation in the program is mandatory. Attendance at the Workcamp is voluntary, but whoever decides to participate is expected to really participate.

In the end it will be clear which of the boys has enough determination to enter into our therapeutic communal life-training program—to experience for six months the school of life and humanity, to sense God's love and to learn discipline, without drugs, alcohol, nicotine. We will structure the transition from Workcamp into the Onesimo program as seamlessly as possible, so that no drug consumption can interfere.

Letter from Manila

November 6, 1996. All the suitcases are packed, the children are asleep, and we are ready to drive back to Manila tomorrow morning. We have had a wonderful time by the sea with the children and my mother. Chris was busy for two weeks with the twenty-five boys who are attempting the start of a new, drug-free life here in Camp Rock. Thanks to the support of my mother, I could allow Chris as much freedom as necessary for this intense time. She will fly back to Switzerland on the day after tomorrow, into the cold!

Now I'm looking forward to being with Chris again, after almost three weeks. In the last couple of weeks I have again had time for my hobbies! I go swimming regularly and I sew—partly simply for myself, but once a week also with the girls in the neighborhood.

The nine months until our vacation at home next summer will now fly by. Isabel knows that she will soon travel to Switzerland and, we hope, see snow for the first time! When she grows up, Daddy will take her with him to do some mountain climbing. She learned many new Swiss-German words from my mother. Nonetheless, she usually speaks Tagalog, ever more fluently. Now and again—exactly at the right moment—she says: "Well, yeah!"

Isabel has many friends, is spoiled by the Filipinos, and in contrast to the slum children, of course, has a very diverse life. Above all, she loves flowers, dolphins, cartoons on television, painting with watercolors. . . . Her most frequent question at the moment is, "Bakit?" That means, "why?" Or "what's going on?" She actually knows many words in all three languages.

Noel is now nine months old. He has four teeth, and the most painful toothaches are over. He crawls very fast and is beginning to try to stand up. Therefore, caring for him is becoming more of a challenge.

Warm Regards, Christine

Beginning of the Communal Organization

The Workcamp is over. It was tough. The group consisted of a tremendously wild crowd of twenty-five teenagers and young adults from different (in part, feuding) street gangs. In the beginning I constantly had the feeling that I was sitting on a live bomb! Without demanding uncompromising adherence to the rules, we leaders wouldn't have had a chance.

It proved to be sensible at first to give some of the boys three days until they could actually take part in all the activities. Such exceptions were based on concern for the heavily addicted, who at the beginning often suffered from headaches, indisposition, and lack of motivation. There were exactly two medications available to treat the side effects of withdrawal: headache pills, as well as discussions and prayers with the leaders.

Each of us eight coworkers were to guide three participants, a very serious responsibility with clear stipulations, such as a daily prayer for intercession, for example, and at a minimum, one personal conversation with each individual, plus the requirement to keep an eye on them constantly. The manual work in the mornings was important to us: The participants were to learn that effort and exertion are worthwhile and bring satisfaction.

The evenings were very moving: We motivated the boys to talk about their lives. Those who couldn't do that were encouraged to draw their lifeline and to indicate special occurrences or impressions with signs and symbols. It was astounding how these rough and ready fellows opened up within the framework of a secure group. Telling their stories with tears in their eyes was not unusual. And again and again it was a prayer, individually delivered loudly and clearly, that transformed this time into a holy moment. Even weeks later, several boys reported that they encountered Jesus, that is, God, at such a moment and had felt an inner strength they had not known before.

A highpoint of the Workcamp was the two-day climb on Malasimbo, a prominent mountain visible from everywhere, which was covered with the last bit of rain forest on the island. Above all, the overnight stay in the open, under a bright tropical sky full of stars, following an earlier campfire, was an overpowering experience of nature and gave the participants another opportunity to open their lives to others.

An accounting of the Workcamps: Four boys had to be sent home early because of discipline problems. Once it was a dangerous fight without any possibility of reconciliation, another time it was simply repetitive cigarette consumption. Of the twenty-one boys that finished the Workcamp, we accepted nine into our communal program in Frisco. Among them are our seven boys from the mountain of rubbish in Payatas, as well as a boy from Potrero and one additional from the impoverished quarter, Paho. They are sufficiently motivated, and their desire for change is most honest. We encouraged the remaining twelve to visit us in Manila and, if necessary and possible, perhaps enter the Onesimo program later.

Now our charges have moved into Onesimo house and we will try to anchor this communal organization as firmly as possible. I am not only grateful for the good team, but also that in the meantime we are again officially full members of Servants in Manila. There are two primary reasons for this: For one, the Australian team leader who was an important factor in our exclusion, was sent home. For another, Charles and Rita Ringma, the house parents of the Servants house strongly and energetically supported us with determination, and discussed the situation with the leaders of Servants Switzerland, Stephan and Monika Thiel. They also convinced the international leadership team to reinstate us.

So we are Servants again. We pursue our Onesimo ministry besides and are answerable for our projects and accountable for them to the leadership of Onesimo. We are happy though about the spiritual support of the Servants team of Manila.

Learning to Live Together

Camp Rock has become habitable. The house is renovated, plumbing and electrical conduits have been laid, a solid guard kiosk has been built. We have already planned a series of one-week camps this year for teenagers from ten slums. They may become a focal point in our work with young people. We especially want to train young people to the point that they can work with us as leaders of small groups from time to time. Perhaps we can place our Onesimo students in logistical positions or even as small group leaders. In all of this, we profit from our own years of experience in CVJM in Switzerland and from the some remarkable Christian youth program's in New Zealand.* The program module is intended to empower young people not only to consume but also to be producers themselves.

Our therapeutic communal organization is challenging and heartening at the same time. The nine teenagers and four coworkers are all still fully engaged. Often enough, we tremble and become anxious about individuals who suddenly, without any obvious reason, opt out, no longer able to tolerate the pressure of discipline and commitment, and want to pull away. Our coworkers have little experience and are instructed to learn from me how one steps in and takes action in an argument (where my forthright Swiss manner naturally comes to the fore). Participants and coworkers have felt hurt by me more than once; apologizing to them later in public has made our relationship on equal terms and credible, however.

The day in the communal life group is clearly structured: morning devotions; breakfast; sports; clean-up; washing; water fetching; shopping; cooking; eating; siesta. In the afternoon there is either volunteer work in the neighborhood, the preparation for an evening outreach effort in the streets, or reading, writing, and arithmetic with a teacher who comes to us. After the evening meal we visit children and youths on the street, armed mostly with sandwiches, fruit juice, and guitar. Or we watch TV or play games. Sometimes we organize a movie night. Life in the community is free. Nevertheless, everyone must help with all of the work; nobody gets pocket money.

Before going to sleep, there is always an "Evening Round," with a common prayer for one another. Here we learn to reflect and to live consciously, instead of simply existing. There is much to discuss—our house is cramped, conflicts are unavoidable. During the Round, we can resolve arguments verbally rather

---

* Cf Lloyd Martin, The Invisible Table: Perspectives on Youthwork in New Zealand (Dunmore Press, 2002)

than with fists. More than once during the day a fight has erupted and reflexively, someone reached for the kitchen knife. In the evening we can then consciously practice reconciliation visible to everyone—again and again. These Evening Rounds are binding and one of the most important elements in the rehabilitation of the young people. There are some very emotional moments, in which we sense God's presence and a calmness comes over us, which almost always accompanies me personally into a peaceful sleep.

The potential for violence in the young men sometimes appears completely without warning. Once after a movie outing together, we wanted to return home in a rented minivan, but couldn't get out of the parking garage because a bus was blocking the exit. Sounding the horn brought no response; the driver was calmly waiting for passengers. After several minutes of patient waiting, I shouted at the driver that he should finally get out of our way. No reaction. Suddenly all the doors of our van flew open, and my Onesimo boys ran to the bus, armed with steel keys, lifting jacks, and other instruments to inflict blows. My blood ran hot and cold, and I rushed up behind them, shouting that they should come back. Attracted by the noise, the police quickly appeared. Somehow I managed to pacify the defenders of the law, and to get my team back into our van, where I read them the riot act. In that evening's Round, we had a lot to talk about.

Our buddy system has proven to be central: Nobody is to leave the house alone. A coworker or another participant should always go along. Thus the boys support one another to keep from losing momentum, since drugs, alcohol, and girls are easily had in the slum. Support and transparency are important.

Not long ago we determined that the boys may visit their families and friends once a week, naturally accompanied by a coworker. When a boy has the feeling that life with Onesimo consists only of renunciation, renunciation, and renunciation, then a glance at the reality of others is helpful. Such a glimpse moves the profit that he gains through the life lessons he is taught into the proper light.

Twice per week, all the boys in our little house are invited to a common meal. Isabel and Noel contribute much fun and laughter and we all enjoy these meals very much. As people who themselves experience healing from God, we allow ourselves to be used at the same time to pass healing on.

A few weeks ago, we coworkers and participants spent a night outside the city. As we began singing and praying that evening, we were surprised by an unusually strong welling up of feelings that caught us involuntarily and brought us to tears. It was a mixture of regret caused by guilt and a sense of one's own failure and the impact of the realization that God loves us unconditionally.

In one of our coworker Rounds I told the others of my dream of a kind of material commune: To live like the early Christians, all from the same cash box, trusting that there would be enough to cover everyone's needs.

Eyebrows were raised; many wrinkled their brows—and in the next Round they explained the complication in the idea to me: For them, as poor Filipinos, it would be impossible to delineate their own needs from those of their relatives and friends. Their life is interwoven in familiar and other broader relationships, and they are obligated to help all of them with their income, when need is present. They would rather have a self-earned wage for personal use. A longer dependency on Onesimo would thereby also be avoided.

This position corresponded unequivocally to the concepts of our Filipino executive committee which already had determined a wage scale for Onesimo coworkers. So my idea was off the table. I found it regrettable, but appropriate. I am proud that our decision making process was based on a straightforward, open partnership with mutual respect. There are enough NGOs, missions, and churches with an unpleasant distance between *policy-setting* foreign leaders and *performing* Filipino followers.

Two Busses, One Nightmare

I could have tossed the whole miserable kettle of fish. All one can do is cry! What happened?

We're writing at the beginning of March—and the bus project still has not yielded any profits for Onesimo. As a result, I demand from my friend in charge of the enterprise a straightforward accounting—and sure enough: No profit is apparent. My friend twists and turns and speaks of many unexpected expenses as, for example, a little accident. "What kind of accident?" I want to know. A small child tore away from his mother, he says, and was hit by our bus, and lost his life. In such a case in this country, the organization pays the family a sum for pain and suffering in the amount of 15,000 pesos (577 US dollars), even if the driver is not at fault.

I am horrified, particularly because I hadn't been told about this terrible occurrence. I ask my friend who this unfortunate driver might be. He tells me his name, one of his friends. I know him from the neighborhood—he is a notorious alcoholic and one-time criminal, about whom I was never entirely sure if the "one-time" really applied.

Now I blow my top. "How could you make such a bad choice and then keep the apparent consequences secret from me?" I scream at my friend.

"He has thirty years of experience as a chauffeur," he defends himself, "he is the father of one of the Onesimo coworkers, and I wanted to help him. . . ."

The next day Pastor Noel comes to me in despair and says that he has learned from reliable sources that our friend and manager of the project had added a bus for himself some time ago, and was successfully reaping a profit for his own purse. We calculate our outlay: The price of the second Onesimo bus had most probably been enough for two busses. That almost does me in. I have known this man for years. He is one of the few in my environment who has a high school diploma, is multi-talented, and trustworthy. If it had been different, I would not have trusted him with our idea.

On the same evening I call him to account, face to face. He denies everything; it is pure slander, Noel is just jealous. During the discussion it becomes clear to me all at once, however, that I have not just my friend before me, but also a deceiver. And it becomes clear to me that I likely first brought him to temptation to deceive through my trust. As a slum dweller, he has probably also become a victim of his dreams of a better life. I should have listened to Christine who warned me several times that in her opinion, this coworker had problems with the truth. I always explained in response that it was just a matter of differing cultural values.

In the evening I call Harry Roque who is also the president of Onesimo. We call a meeting for the next day. The executive committee advises me unanimously to keep my distance from this situation from now on. I am too close to the manager to remain objective. Now dispassionate minds are needed. They will clarify the situation and undertake the necessary steps.

The shock is deep. This man did not only hurt me personally, he also betrayed Onesimo—actually everything that we stand for and that we want to accomplish.

Letter from Manila

Frisco, March 21, 1997. Dear Ones, we have a difficult time behind us. The breach of trust of our friend is especially hard for Chris to cope with. Pastor Noel and Franklin had to step in and fully take over the bus business in order to save the situation. Thereby, they will not be able to participate in the camps scheduled for the immediate future. But God is seeing to that, too. We have already found other coworkers for several of the camps.

We hope that at the end of April our life will become normal again. Despite all the pressures that burden and despite the never-ending work, Chris is strong. I can't quite imagine how he can cope with everything without becoming very testy or nervous. In our relationship we experience God's grace and help. We stand together in everything and try to carry one another. It's a great gift! Isabel, Noel, Ron, and Jessica do everything with us. Noel feels happy as a clam in the midst of the many children and young people.

Together with Isabel I visited a private Philippine preschool two days ago. Perhaps after our return from our vacation at home, she can be registered there. She says nearly every day that she would like to go to preschool.

Cordially, Christine

Paths to the World of Work

Camp Rock is running incredibly well. The house is being used by a variety of groups that work among the poor. We ourselves have instituted a leadership school with sixty motivated participants as well as four summer leisure programs with a total of 350 children from thirteen slums. Even still, weeks later, we receive encouraging reports from groups and communities about the positive changes in the lives of their young people.

The nine boys from our therapeutic communal living group also helped us efficiently in the camps. They have finished the first six months of their rehabilitation and no one left the program.

"That never happened before," Charles Ringma commented exuberantly. He would know, since he has spent half his life dealing with the rehabilitation of drug-addicted youngsters.

The path into the working world has been more difficult for our boys up to now. We've taken great pains to provide all the necessary papers for the job search for each individual, including residential permits, physician's reports, character references, and the like. Naturally, they can't and don't want to hide their backgrounds as former addicts and street children. Their faces and their tattoos, in part, speak clearly. Through role playing, we practiced attitude discussions so that they would know what to anticipate. For weeks, our boys took to the road daily to find themselves jobs. They came back in the evening tired and frustrated. A picture of distress!

One day Pastor Noel and I ventured out to take on the search for jobs. We spoke with ten heads of personnel and recommended our diligent and highly motivated young men. We promised that in the case of possible problems our Foundation would assume the responsibility. We received seven partly angry, partly friendly rejections. The remaining three consoled us with a later appointment. Noel and I returned home every bit as tired, frustrated, and aggrieved as the boys. This is how it feels when one isn't wanted. Very depressing.

Shortly thereafter a Coca Cola factory hired our entire group. Super! On the first workday, there was literally no quitting time: Our boys were to haul boxes deep into the night, without special wages. The foremen were paid for each box, according to what we could tally. On the second day, we discontinued this practice.

A few weeks later the turning point occurred and in various areas at the same time. We had the opportunity to sell the older of our two buses. With the proceeds we could not only pay off the new bus, which ran remarkably well, but we could also purchase two houses in the rubble slum, Payatas. In one of them, three of our boys together with our coworkers Arnold and William, run a small tire repair and welding workshop as well as a little pig-breeding business. A potential mother sow is avidly being fed left overs from the refuse heap. In the other house, Pastor Jun Arizala leads our new second Onesimo house community.

For two other boys, we furnished a sandal workshop in Frisco. Their master-teacher is my old friend and ex-gangster Rico from Potrero. Yet two other protégés were placed in a factory. John, the previous head of the Payatas group, has begun a course of study to become an auto mechanic. With two exceptions, all of them continue to live in our communal quarters.

In the meantime, we came into a third communal living situation relatively unexpectedly: Joshua Palma took part in a leisure program at Camp Rock, with sixty children from the improvised shelters of the evacuated scavengers. Since then, a core group of about fifteen youths have been meeting with him for discussion, prayer, Bible reading, and eating. Joshua asked us to support him—and so we now have a third communal living establishment in Tondo, the largest slum in Manila, with Joshua as the house father.

Over the last few weeks we have had a number of discussions with my "friend," the manager of the bus enterprise, during which further unpleasant stories saw the light of day. He consistently denied everything, until the claim could be substantiated with evidence. Then he wailed and begged for forgiveness. He left only when our attorney, Harry, threatened him with indictment and prison. I have seldom been so sad in my entire life. I am so infinitely grateful to Christine, the executive committee, all my friends, and especially our honest and conscientious Noel Gabaldon for their understanding and support during this time. To be betrayed is among the worst that can happen to a person.

Three weeks later we are sitting on the hard wooden benches in the small chapel in Frisco and listen with brimming eyes to the farewell song of our friends. In a few days, just after three years in the slum, we will depart for Switzerland for six months. So many friends are sitting here, so many developments and stories!

Leaving Ron and Jessica, who have lived with us such a long time, is like a separation within a family. Noel and Isabel will miss them very much. "Don't be afraid," says Isabel. "We'll come back soon and will bring you flowers and snow."

Letters from Manila

January 1998. A wonderful half year in Switzerland lies behind us. Swiss mountains, Swiss amenities, autumn woods. At the same time, overwhelming interest and support for our work, not only from our families and friends, but also from many church congregations, youth groups, and home circles in which we have an opportunity to report on what we are doing.

During the entire six months the news from Pastor Noel and Pastor Joshua from Tondo, Frisco, and Payatas cheered us. Despite our absence, our coworkers carried out the leadership training in March/April during the big summer leisure program. Huge! Evidence of trusting in God, trusting in self and being proactive, all values that we try to further through our example and on the basis of the Bible.

Our "little Filipino" Noel was in Switzerland for the first time! We hope that the children will more or less manage the return to slum life. In six months, Isabel is to enter preschool—in the Philippines, reading and writing already begins at age four or five.

After landing at the Ninoy Aquino International Airport, the familiar scent of Manila envelopes me. At customs, Western efficiency has definitely come to an end—everything again becomes complicated and annoying. First I get angry. Then I have to recall that all the hindrances have their reason, that many people here fight every day to survive, and that it's actually amazing how much does indeed work.

The noise, dirt, stench, and heat of this gigantic city transpose me into a state of shock. I came back here voluntarily? In my memory much was more positive and more beautiful. The first days in the Servants house I feel as if I am lame.

A ray of light are our visits to the communities in Frisco and Tondo. The biggest news however, still awaits us: The coworkers find that we are needed more in Payatas, at Onesimo's second training center, than in Frisco. It all sounds convincing to Chris and me, but to move there is asking a lot, even of a slum family. We discuss, pray . . . and slowly become amenable to the thought.

Manila, March 5, 1998. *Tomorrow we will finally move into a little house in Payatas. The layout is approximately 13 feet x 13 feet, with two floors. Upstairs we have created three (!) little rooms out of this expanse, where we and the children sleep. On the lower floor is the kitchen, with dining table, refrigerator, and a daybed for visitors. In the bath/toilet, one can hardly turn around. In front of the house, we have a small, enclosed veranda and a Jackfruit tree that provides shade. Next to the kitchen, from which one door leads outside, we have our open pigsties. The house next door (about three feet from ours) is occupied by a group of Onesimo boys.*

I am very happy although I am aware that in Payatas we will be living far away from the inner city and from all other missionaries. Boredom will also become a topic. Two, three houses away, there is a small, basic Christian community meeting in a chapel and a slum kindergarten. About 300 feet from our house, the enormous garbage dump site of Payatas begins.

Last week someone off-loaded twelve containers of a highly poisonous substance onto the rubble heap, almost in front of our shack. Our boys had to close all the windows. Then the police became involved and removed it all. I don't want to know where the material then landed—but it made headlines in the newspaper.

Love, Christine

The Vultures of Payatas

"Thus you will recognize the Redeemer of the world: He lies wrapped in swaddling clothes in a manger for animals . . . ," I read in the Gospel of St. Luke. The grotesque sentence fits nicely into this rubbish-heap settlement.

About 4:00 a.m., the trucks' diesel motors are turned on again and again, and with a loud howling noise, empty their filthy exhaust pipes directly onto our little house. But what can one do? If the wind from the pile of rubble turns in our direction, we'll be fogged in by a sweetly-rotten garbage odor anyway. Recently

Christine and I awoke at the same time. There was a horrid stench. At first we felt only a burning in our throats, but then we had to fight feelings of nausea. Let's hope that these clouds of smoke have no serious health implications.

Our new place of residence remains a challenge. Isabel sometimes cries in the evenings because she misses her cousins and friends in Switzerland; furthermore, she complains that she is laughed at by the others because she no longer speaks Tagalog. Noel has to be watched constantly outside the house, because the children's playground is located on a field littered with trash and shards of glass.

And yet, strangely, despite everything, we slowly begin to feel well here. When the wind blows from the "good direction," that is, from the nature preserve where the reservoir with the drinking water for Manila lies, we find the climate more bearable than in the inner city Frisco slum. Payatas is a so-called "shantytown," a very large slum settlement of individual shacks at the edge of the city, with many trees. We even have a view of the nearby hills of Montalban, the adjacent province. But on the same plane as our house, we have the rubbish heap!

Today I accompany the morning shift to pick garbage. At five o'clock in the morning, I shuffle along behind Marcello and John up the mountain of rubbish, with rubber boots on my feet and a steel awl with a hook—my first experience as a "carrion vulture." I am familiar with early morning departures when it's still almost dark from mountain climbing in Switzerland—except there the mountains are different. . . .

I try to act as if tripping through the trash were the most normal thing in the world. There are also a couple of hundred others that have resigned themselves to this repugnant, demeaning work. In my case it concerns only feed for our pigs; two or three hours in the early morning every day are enough. Most of the others have to tramp through the biting stench all day, and sometimes also at night, with miner's lamps on their foreheads.

At the beginning I stand around somewhat helplessly and let myself suffer the smirks of the other people. I smile in return. They look at me and ask themselves what this Amerikano has lost here. Then they turn back to the garbage.

Marcello and John have developed a kind of sensor to determine where the best food scraps can be found. The most disgusting aspect occurs after the tearing open of the bags—the digging through the stinking rubbish—with bare hands, otherwise one doesn't have the right "feel." Namely, foil or plastic would not be good for our pigs. Thereby, one naturally encounters viscous things like dirty diapers, decayed rats, feces packed in paper or plastic bags. Eighty percent of the poor in Payatas don't have a water closet of their own. Their alternative: newspaper or plastic bags. Odors of decay of innards almost take one's breath away. They can be found primarily in market bags, in which one can otherwise also fish for relatively well-preserved vegetables.

One has to be careful during this process to avoid inadvertently digging in a pile that already belongs to a superior garbage picker. The market economy here has its own rules. If someone has some money, he buys an entire truck's contents from the trash collection depot syndicate. If I want to dig around in that pile, I have to strike a deal with its new owner. That corresponds apparently with Marcellos's and John's method: While they diligently keep looking for old food, they also gather glass, aluminum, and good plastic in a separate basket. With this they pay for their burrowing rights to the "owner" of the pile.

It was my good fortune that a jolly woman took pity on me and explained what was appropriate for pigs and how I should best proceed. And then a joyful shout: "Oh, that's the truck from the Hilton Hotel. There's good food in it!" And away she went.

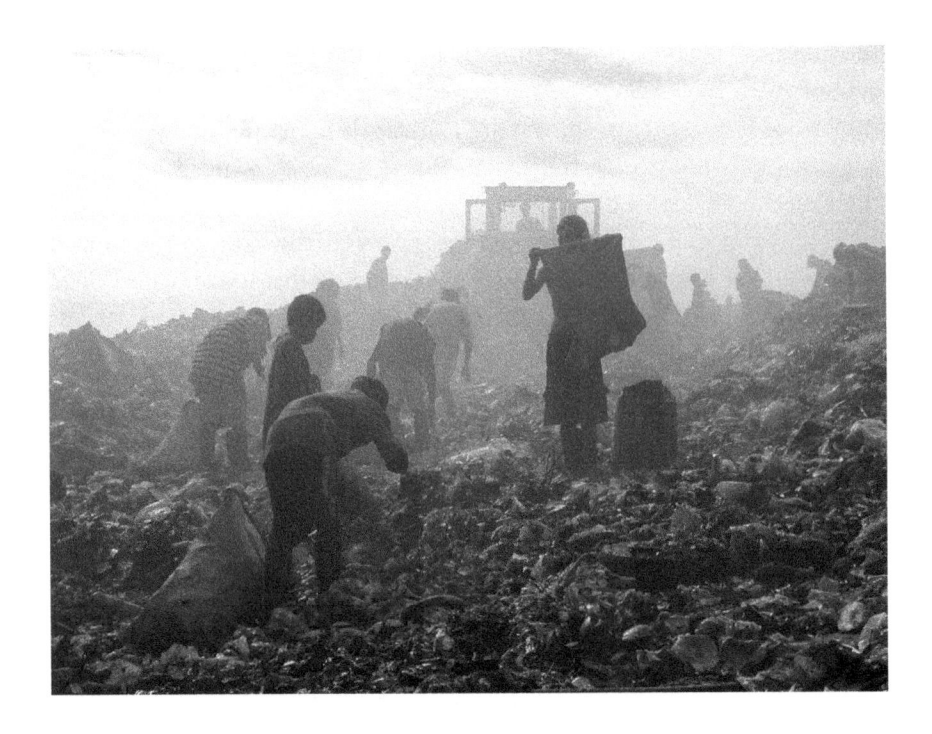

At 5:00 a.m., I shuffle up the mountain of rubble, rubber boots on my feet and a steel awl with a hook in my hand. My first experience as a "scavenger."

Above all, it is children, teenagers, and aged people who collect here. I also meet up with a few well-groomed mothers and hale and hearty men from our neighborhood. And Ate Viki, the wife of the pastor of the small Christian congregation next door. I imagine how rich Christians in air conditioned, expensive-style buildings with the most modern music systems praise the Lord, while their siblings in faith in the same city, daily burrow in rubbish in order to survive. The stable in Bethlehem was also not air conditioned. . . .

On the way home, in an open shack, I come across a child's coffin. It's a picture of everyday life—fifty percent of the children here are not well—or undernourished. I stop in for a moment, look around and meet the sad eyes of a pretty, already somewhat bigger teenage girl. "My little brother lies in the coffin—he is only six months old," she answers my questioning glance.

In the evening I visit the family again. Marisa, the emaciated mother with a worn-out face, explains to me that the father is drunk. Everything is so difficult, she says. He was the eighth child and had asthma. But her oldest son has also already died in an accident. "Look at him," she urges me, "he sleeps so peacefully."

"Nanay," I stammer somewhat awkwardly, "your fate moves me very much. I myself am the father of small children. I would like to express my sympathy." Then I put some money in the empty tin, which stands as a collection box next to the little corpse, according to tradition. The burial costs run approximately 6,000 *pesos,* a small fortune for these people. The vicious cycle of debt and misery spins ever further. I quietly pronounce God's blessing on the tired mother. I don't have more and at this point it would perhaps be inappropriate.

Letter from Manila

Manila, March 31, 1998. Yesterday the well in front of the house was finished. In three weeks, five to six men dug a 120 foot deep hole with the most primitive tools. Now the water is being brought to the surface with a pump. Until now we have had only brown water from old wells in the neighborhood. Since the new well is located directly next to the house, we no longer have to carry water into the house a kettle at a time, but rather we can fill the large plastic barrel in the toilet with a hose. Super!

We are the subject of conversation everywhere in Payatas. Apparently, among the 300,000 inhabitants, we are the only foreigners. We have, however, made a few new friends, but I still find life to be a fight for survival and often feel insecure and threatened. And yet, slowly, the conviction returns that it is important to be here above all. Again and again, I experience the Filipinos, whether poor or rich, as enormously helpful and generous. I'd like to be re-infected by that, and in a small way—according to my potential—be there for other people the way Jesus has charged me to be.

We go swimming every week in a pool that is approximately a half hour away. I try to find a young person in the area with a motorcycle with a sidecar who can drive me there with the children. Each time it's an adventure!

With love, Your Christine

An Easter Experience

A good four weeks ago we received a surprise visit from India: Mercy and Wolfgang Simson with their two children spent a week's vacation on "our" beach in Camp Rock. Wolfgang is originally from the same Church congregation in Basel (EGB) as we. He works for the DAWN movement (Discipling a Whole Nation) and as a missionary and networker visiting the Middle East, Asia, and Europe. It was a wonderful surprise for us to have such trusted friends with us suddenly.

Wolfgang reported in his enthusiastic way about a new movement of house churches: Small neighborhood churches led by lay people, that split into two as soon as they have about twenty participants. No expense for theological education opportunities, building projects, music provisions, and complicated leadership structures—simply people, who share their entire life every day and thereby pray to God—a kind of reliving the early Church of the time before Emperor Constantine.

I was listening to Wolfgang only with one ear, since that week at Camp Rock I was intensely occupied with planning the next leisure activities program

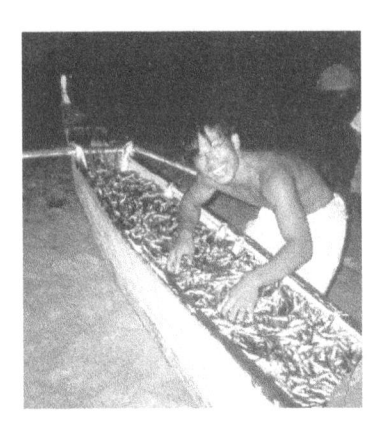

What then happened was fun, surprising, and indescribable fishermen's good fortune.

for 625 participants. But then came Easter Saturday. Christine and I strolled to a nearby restaurant to allow the day to ring out with a cool drink. The white sand, the palms, and the broad sea glistened in the silver light of the full moon. The splashing of small waves emphasized the warm, tropical silence. Even the usual chugging of the fishing boats was missing—there are no fish to be caught during a full moon; everyone here knows that.

Meanwhile, our Onesimo boys sat on the beach, played the guitar, and chatted. Suddenly they discovered a large dark shadow in the water, immediately at their feet. "Look everybody, it's a swarm of fish," one of them called out. The boys sprang up, found an old mosquito net nearby and, in high spirits, ran into the water with it. What then happened was fun, surprise, and indescribable fishermen's good fortune: The boys stood hip deep in the water, surrounded by thousands of small leaping fish. With the help of the mosquito net, but also with bare hands and tubs that they brought down for the purpose, they filled a fishing boat lying on the beach up to its rim, and in addition, all the available containers in Camp Rock.

We took the greater part of the fish to the market during the night and sold them for a nice profit. There had to have been several thousand fishes; we playfully claimed to top the biblical miracle of the 153 fish with ours on Easter morning. During the full moon, there are no fishes to be caught—everyone here knows that . . . a miracle!

A few hours later, on Easter morning, there was delicious grilled fish for breakfast. Excitedly, we read chapter 21 of the Gospel of St. John, where it is described how the newly risen surprises his disciples with a "fish breakfast": "Come and breakfast."

First we look at each other silently. Then Ate Josy, our "mother" and chief cook says: "Jesus lives!"

On the same morning, the Simsons say goodbye to us. "There's something else," Wolfgang remarks at the last minute. "That there were small and many fishes refers to the fact that many small people are implicated. And that it was an old mosquito net means that it happened in an extraordinary way. And be prepared, it will happen fast and without great effort."

Workcamp and the Everyday

June 1998. Tomorrow Workcamp begins at Camp Rock. It serves as bridge and entry for our garbage pickers and street kids into the communal living facilities of Onesimo. We wait with pounding hearts at the agreed-upon meeting place, but none of the destitute boys from the dump site appear. For them the step is apparently too big, the shame, the insecurity, of being together with non-garbage pickers.

We start out to look for them. Our coworker John, the former gang leader, leads us through the falling dusk to the black, slimy mountain of rubbish, sure of his destination. One has to know the paths here so as not to become stuck in the disgusting swamp or lose one's way.

Suddenly we stand in our rubber boots and with wobbly knees in front of a half destroyed shanty hut with skull graffiti at the entrance. About ten boys and young men sit or lie around a little fire on which a soup bubbles. They are filthy and wrapped in rags. Most of them sniff at bags of glue. Half-grown-up boys and girls lie in the semi-darkness, intertwined with one another, some staring into emptiness with wide open eyes.

John knows Allen, the leader of the group, from before. He is thin as a rake, and has restless and penetrating eyes. We speak about Onesimo, about the camp, about the boys who actually wanted to come but had not appeared at the meeting point. John talks about his experiences.

Six boys get ready to come with us, all of them in front of Allen! Perhaps it's only the expectation of a real meal that moves them to follow us. But my heart is beating with happiness. I sincerely prayed for such a miracle. We head to Onesimo house. The boys clearly enjoy the fresh water, the soap, the steaming rice with large pieces of meat.

The next morning it's off the Camp Rock. We ride in the mini-bus that our friends in the OJC in Reichelsheim financed for us. The boys look comical—all of them are wearing my T-shirts that are several sizes too large. In Cubao some additional young people join in; they were drummed up by friends of Help International CMC (Christian Missionary Community), based in Lüdenscheid, Germany for our Camp. On the ferry, there will still be other participants, and coworkers from Tondo will join us.

We get to know the twenty teenagers a little during the first few days. They are completely unpredictable. There is Jimmy, for example, seventeen-years-old, pretty undernourished, with an infected wound on his right shin bone. His mother works in a nightclub; he doesn't know his father. He ran away because his mother's boyfriend constantly molested him. He has already been living in the asphalt jungle of the large metropolis and recruits customers for group taxis. If he is able to assemble a sufficient number, he earns enough to eat, sometimes even to go to a movie. Several times, Jimmy tried to save a little, but the few *pesos* were regularly stolen from him, even when he hid the money in his underpants. Sometimes he is tortured by people. Once they set his bare feet on fire with newspaper, as he slept on the sidewalk. When it gets very tight financially, he sells himself to men for sex. But actually he hates that.

While we listen to the stories of the many boys at camp—stories that take one's breath away—Christine holds the line at home:

It is half past eleven in the morning. "Bayang magiliw . . ." With her right hand on her heart and hollow cross, Isabel sings the Philippine national anthem in the small preschool next door. Then she says a pledge of allegiance with the other children in the choir to "her Fatherland," the Philippines, and anticipating praise, behaves according to that which her parents, teachers, and leaders tell her. The many teachers working in the preschools of the impoverished settlements have at most a minimal education and practically no resources. Therefore teaching is limited to pronunciation and repetition, copying, and singing. And that in rooms far too small, under a hot tin roof. Isabel's school bag is filled with books and notebooks for entries and homework. Language instruction consists of Tagalog, which she again speaks fluently. In reading and writing, English takes precedence.

Yesterday we avoided a tragedy by a hair's breadth. Jonathan, Nar, Romeo, Bic, Allen, and Erwin from the drug gang at the rubble mountain hate another participant from Tondo. Whatever the reason, the gang decided to kill him with shovels and then run away to Manila. "Somehow" something interfered.

Since it's too hot outside, I spend a lot of time with the children in the dark lower floor of our slum shack. Drawing, playing with Legos, looking at little books and videos; for the children, the days are often too short. For me, boredom sneaks in now and again, when I don't get out of Payatas at times. Visits and excursions include burdensome trips however; mile-long traffic jams in tropical heat and in exhaust fumes, squeezed between sweating fellow travelers. . . . I am glad when Chris is here again. I pray that it goes well with these wild boys. Chris carries an immense responsibility.

We have discovered that Bic, a street kid, has a large machete with him, even at night. He needs it because Allen has a hidden axe with him. A war prevails between the two. We tried to calm Bic and to call upon him to make peace, but he became more agitated and stubborn. Determined, we prayed to Jesus, whom the Bible calls the "Prince of Peace." Bic became calm before our eyes and was then even ready to speak with Allen. After another prayer they shook hands and asked one another for forgiveness. If these aren't miracles, what is?

Isabel has made a good beginning. Noel has gone along quite a few times and has reverently sat next to Isabel on the school bench. The teacher tolerates this happily. The fat little Amerikano draws a smile everywhere, and everyone likes to pinch his cheek, which he doesn't appreciate at all. He is quite social, however, and also already speaks quite a bit of Tagalog.

Today we returned from a two-day "mountain trip,"—A luminous morning between the shrubs of a kind of grass terrace, 1,200 feet above the South China Sea. We sat—still somewhat stiff from the night in the open air—with steaming cups of coffee in our hands. First we laughed at a couple of jokes. Then it became quiet and we enjoyed the fresh breeze, which felt so good together with the first rays of the sun.

One of us began to pray and invited us also to offer a prayer of gratitude to the Creator of this splendor. Another actually followed another with timid, stammering, but nonetheless determined sentences. I am now still moved by the experience. That is not an acquired religiosity. That is the breaking out of a long buried relationship to God; the awakening desire for home with the father.

Noel is a "people person." He wants to know who is going where, who's going to come along, when we will leave, what belongs to whom and so forth. Isabel is much more objective. I noticed this again just recently: We both are on the way home to Payatas and pass the large market in the main street of Payatas. A pig is just in the process of being dismembered on a table; the head and the entrails are lying adjacent. Isabel goes right up to it with great curiosity, watches for a while and says cooly: "Now I finally know what a pig looks like inside."

At the end of the two-week Workcamp the decision is made which boys can enter the Onesimo training program. The offer is extended even for Isko and Resty. But they decline. The temptation of unbridled "freedom" on the street is stronger. With heavy hearts we let them move on.

September Days

I am happy about Isko and Resty. A few weeks ago they stood in front of our Onesimo center in Payatas and excitedly told us that they were ready to enter the communal living program. "Now I'm sick of the streets!", Isko said, and showed me a fresh knife wound on his back. Resty, since the Workcamp, had been reading his new Bible on the sidewalk where he lived and was tormented and laughed at. Now he also has found a new home with us.

We have sold the bus. Although five people were employed as a result of this project and it earned a small monthly profit for Onesimo, it was not worthwhile. The leadership is looking around for better profit-making ventures.

On Sunday evening, Nora appeared at our front door, with a typical Philippine smile on her beautiful face. She is now eighteen-years-old, the mother of the sweet Rixy, and since three weeks ago, a widow. Her husband, a garbage picker and also hardly beyond his teenage years, was stabbed in his sleep. Revenge as a result of an old quarrel, according to the neighbors.

"Tomorrow I could begin working as a housemaid for a rich family, but what would I do with my Rixy?" Nora is relatively new in our slum and hardly trusts her neighbors. We take her, with her problem that has now also become our problem, to a good family in the local church community. There we discuss various possibilities and offer to take the sweet baby for the first few days ourselves.

On Monday afternoons, four older coworkers and I meet regularly with Annabel Manalo, a trained psychologist. She helps us to reflect and to handle ourselves, our experiences, and those entrusted to us.. To spend time debriefing with her is always a real pleasure!

After supper the meeting continues: we pray, make plans, exchange information. One of the points for today's discussion is weighty: The newly selected parliamentary deputy, Dingh, would like us to open a rehabilitation center for youths in his city, Pasay. Our conversation last week appears to have influenced him. Our attorney, Harry Roque, a trusted friend of Dingh, has offered to provide for us without cost a 3,300 square foot piece of land with a half-destroyed two-story house, in the middle of an indigent quarter. Naturally we're enthused but also alarmed at the same time. With our three existing centers, we're already close to our capacity in terms of personnel. We'll have to postpone the decision and listen to God: first, *if* and then *how* and *when*.

On Tuesday Christine meets with the wife of a coworker whose marriage is in dangerous crisis. We feel our own helplessness in this conflict, but are determined to support both parties without choosing sides. If only they don't let go of God's hand!

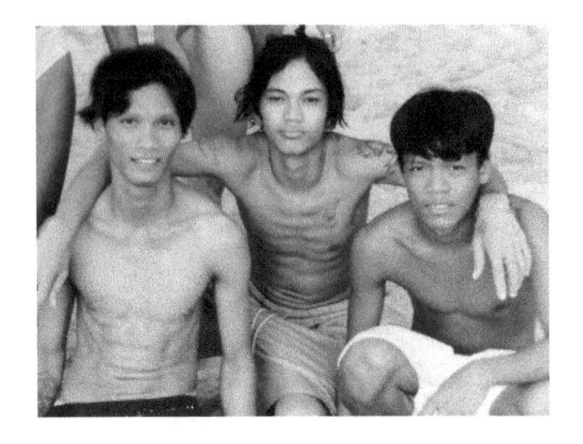

Gerald (middle), one of the wild boys, fresh from the street.

On Wednesday, the twenty-year-old Gerald packs his three possessions in a plastic sack and wants to leave the communal living facility: "I don't belong here, I'll never change."

We tell him that he has changed immensely already: "You've been free of drugs, thievery, and pimping for three months! We're simply not going to let you go." An hour-long "battle" ensues, with discussion and prayer. Gerald finally unpacks his things again. Who knows, for how long.

On Thursday, Berardo moves in, for a few days or perhaps weeks. The starving glue sniffer is fifteen, has the body of a ten-year-old, however, almost black skin and large, sad eyes. We simply couldn't leave him behind in the rubbish yesterday evening at our weekly visit to the trash-heap gang. He has a fever and he can't move his right hand because of a large infected wound. Almost without a will of his own, he allowed us to lead him away. No word has passed his lips yet. Shame, devoid of feelings, or brain damage—that has yet to be determined.

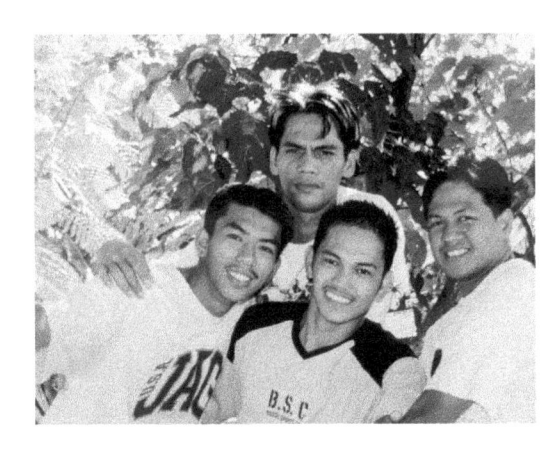

Gerald, a few months later, in the residential community

On Friday Gerald tells me that he is plagued by voices that pull him away from us. I advise taking him to Dr. Randy for an appointment, our Filipino friend who is a professional psychiatrist and also on the Board of Onesimo. In addition, Cory comes by for a short visit. She is a professor at a theological institute and supports our work. She asks if she may bring a visitor from the United States to see us next week. At this occasion we would also meet two other pastors from Payatas, which is important for our networking locally.

On Saturday, Pastor Jun Arizala organizes the promised day off. We have too few companion guides so not everyone can go. This affects the mood. Romeo has wanted to visit his father for a long time. He is serving a life sentence in the high security prison in Muntinlupa. So far a visit hasn't worked out—the trip there and back takes about five hours, the visit regulations are complicated.

At the end of this week we take time out for a family excursion. We have a choice of a shopping center with a playground, a swimming pool, or a city park with horses and roller skating. It isn't quite so hot any longer, so we head to the city park. We have to be back in the early afternoon, however, or we'll get stuck in the evening's gridlock.

In the following week, Dr. Randy calls and advises me urgently to allow Gerald to return to the street: "He is psychotic. He hears voices who order him to kill himself or people at Onesimo. The boy is dangerous."

I am thunderstruck. How often we have prayed for healing and deliverance! May I not consider it a miracle that for two months such a wild "animal" has been leading such an orderly life with us? I speak with Gerald, and he agrees that we speak openly in the group about his condition and about Randy's recommendation. After discussion and prayer the group unanimously decides that Gerald can stay despite the risk.

Randy acquiesces—with the stipulation that Gerald agrees to be treated with medication and attends talk-therapy sessions weekly.

The eighteen-year-old Nora has now found a neighbor who watches Rixy. She will share her wages with her. And Bernardo is here again, after having disappeared for two days. His wound healed quickly, thanks to antibiotics, and he has become somewhat more talkative. We have invited him to become a committed Onesimo participant and have explained the regulations to him. He is considering it.

"I didn't think that he would hurt me"

A few weeks ago I heard noise in front of our shack and suddenly Jessica stands in front of me: "Something has happened to Mylene—come quickly...."

Outside the small, dirty girl from the neighborhood cowers—she is twelve-years-old. "A... A... Arol w... was always so nice to us, I never... tho... tho ... thought that he would hurt me...." Mylene sobs, and is actually shaking.

Carefully I put my arm around her narrow shoulders and search for eye contact with those that had hurried over. *Do something, she is a child from your neighborhood*, I think, but don't say aloud.

"She deserves it, she is a little tramp and belongs to the glue sniffers," says one of the neighbors and walks away. The contempt in his voice almost hurts me physically. The other onlookers also leave. Gently we nudge Mylene into our home. Here she can cry without embarrassment for a good long time. Gratefully, she then takes a bath and eats something.

Mylene belongs to the group of girls who again and again come to us for a meal, a bath, or simply to stop by. She has also taken part in Jessica's Bible-discussion Circle. Although the girls typically have a family, they live in self-constructed shacks on the rubbish heap. They are glue or meth addicted.

We also know Arol. Sober, the eighteen-year-old is an amiable young man. He actually lived with us in the Center for a few weeks, but had become drunk at every opportunity and then became very aggressive. One day he wanted to hide from the police at Onesimo because he had stabbed another boy in a fight. It's not always clear here if one can trust the police. In his case we saw little reason to protect him from the police, and advised that we would accompany him to the station and stand by his side with an attorney. He rejected our offer and disappeared.

Mylene spends the night with us and leaves the next morning. Two days later she is again sexually attacked by Arol. This time Mylene's fifteen-year-old sister, Jane, comes between them and Arol stabs her in the chest. Neighbors get her to the hospital in time. In the following weeks, the two sisters visit us often. Christine and Jessica take care of them; I remove the stitches from Jane's stab wound. Jessica, encouraged by us, accompanies their mother to the police, to accuse Arol.

Two weeks later, Arol reappears. I worry about the children in the neighborhood and about Isabel. I ask Jessica to alert the police that Arol has returned. For two weeks, Jessica finds reasons to postpone the walk to the police station, and finally admits she is afraid of Arol's vengeance. "If they find out who is responsible for accusing Arol...."

On Saturday evening, under cover of darkness, Jessica and I undertake a search for Mylene's family's shack. For almost a half an hour, I follow Jessica in a rainy drizzle through narrow, slimy slum alleys, along the rusty edges of the corrugated tin roofs that often project into our path exactly at my head height. We find a wretched little hut, and in the light of a miserable oil lamp, find four small children sleeping on straw mats, with the mother nearby. Four little ones, two teenagers, no husband....

The mother agrees to come along, and soon we're stumbling through the starless night.

In the white-washed, sterile room of the police station three bored men dressed in civilian clothes are hanging around on plastic stools. On an old desk lies a large-caliber shot gun, next to which cigarette stubs emit smoke out of half of a food tin.

"Good evening, we would like to speak with the officer in charge," I say. The man next to the desk raises his eyebrows. "Tell him what happed," I encourage Mylene's mother and Jessica, who stand shyly in the background. Both women make their report.

"Arol is known to us," says the officer in charge. "He stabbed another young man approximately a year ago. You should have come to us immediately, however. If this incident happened more than four weeks ago, we can only apprehend Arol with a court-prescribed warrant for his arrest." Although we three are speaking Tagalog, the officer answers in very broken English. He apparently wants to make an impression. It also makes me angry that he addresses me only, paying no attention to the mother of the victim or Jessica.

"Would you please explain to the two women in their language the particulars of what they now have to do," I ask him politely, which he then does.

"On the fifth floor of the city government building is the office of the public defender for the poor. With his help you can initiate a court proceeding. As soon as we receive the warrant for arrest we can spring into action."

Tired and disappointed we begin to head home. At our leave taking, Mylene's mother assures us that she has friends who would stand by her at court. She willingly accepts a few *pesos*, as transportation money to visit the lawyer, and a little extra. Jessica and I doubt that she will go.

The next day we undertake a Sunday excursion as a family in a mini-bus borrowed from Servants. We return about six o'clock in the evening and park in front of our house in the twilight. About sixty feet away a couple of men are standing together, shouting at each other. An evening argument between drunks, I think. But then the group suddenly becomes physical, and from somewhere a chair flies through the air. *Hopefully none of our boys are a part of this*, flashes through my mind. We delay getting out of the car a little longer. Then I see a figure bent and cowering on the ground, while another figure with a pistol takes aim and shoots. The gun flashes, the bent figure collapses on the asphalt. "Quick, into the house," I scream at Christine, grab Noel under his arm and run. A gun battle often results from a single shot.

A couple of men grab the victim like a wounded animal and throw him onto the metal floor of a Jeepney. Someone scatters some dirt on the little spot of blood on the street. Neighbors stand around in discussion. An unknown soldier on leave is supposed to have been the shooter, someone says; Arol provoked him in his evil way. Arol! "Shoot! Shoot!" he shouted at him.

After half an hour, the police arrives in a rusty Jeep. Five abreast, they march up our street, fingers on the triggers of their guns. The officer in charge from last evening appears to be the boss today, too. I step in front of him from the side. "Hi, Boss; I never thought misfortune would befall Arol so quickly, I say, and look him in the eyes.

"He got what he deserves," he responds callously.

The Jeepney brings the wounded Arol to the government hospital, an hour away. There they cut his stomach open from top to bottom in an emergency operation. The bullet penetrated the body next to the collarbone, past organs necessary for life, shot diagonally downward and remained lodged in the buttocks. It will remain there until Arol has recovered to the point that they can operate again.

With our boys, we arrange a visit- and care-service schedule. His father, newly arrived from the provinces, is happy about occasional relief. After Arol is released from the clinic, we nurse him in the Center for a couple of nights. Of course, first the hospital bill of 2,000 *pesos* must be settled, with money that we "lend" him. We all speak with him about God, Jesus, and the everlasting worth of his life. He also appreciates our praying with him.

Arol would certainly have stayed with us if we hadn't sent him home. We didn't want to use his needy situation to manipulate him into our communal living fellowship. "When you have completely regained your strength and still want to begin a new life with us, our door is open to you," we assured him.

This all happened about a week ago. In the meantime, Arol lives in our neighborhood with his father and a younger brother from the provinces. Occasionally, he drinks or smokes a cigarette. He also consumes crystal meth again, one of our boys told me recently. Whenever I see him, he smiles at me: "Chris, nagbabago na ako...."—Chris, I am already becoming a new man...

Mylene has moved to a province nearby with her family. It is rumored that her older sister, Jane, has an "Asawa" now, a husband. She continues to live as a garbage picker and addict in the rubble. We're glad every time when she comes by to see us, naturally with the constant hope that she will also rise one day with the Risen.

It would be far easier if one could simply distinguish between good and evil. But especially in life with the poor, we often enough have a choice between two bad solutions, causing us to choose the lesser of two evils. In the Philippines, drug trafficking and rape carry the death penalty. The police, however, are heavily involved in these crimes. In order not to lose the trust that the addicts have in us, it is important that we not foster too trusting a relationship with the police. Arol is not only a scoundrel, but also a friend.

Tropical Fever

Now it's November, and since January we have already had 11,209 sick and 202 deceased from dengue fever according to the headlines of our daily newspaper. Actually it's many more—since the poor don't go to the hospital with a fever and therefore don't become part of the statistics. The virus is carried by biting mosquitos. It affects blood coagulation, which can cause uncontrolled bleeding to the point of death. Or people with the fever receive too few liquids and die in fever-shock. Besides the enormous head and limb pain, diarrhea and painful eczema can develop. The daily newspaper reports that the San Lazaro Hospital has 418 dengue patients in stationary care: thirteen were in a state of shock because of internal bleeding, above all children. The bed capacity is oversubscribed by 250 percent—and Christine has been plagued for over a week with fever, pains, and terrible fatigue.

Since I myself and most slum workers have already survived dengue once, we take the illness relatively calmly. Medicinal therapy in the clinic is also limited to pain medications and on the provision of liquids and salt. As long as Christine drinks enough and doesn't want to go to the hospital herself, she is well taken care of in the cool lower story of our corrugated tin shack.

One afternoon Christine's condition worsens dramatically. She can't go to the toilet alone any longer, has no will to speak, drink, or even to live. I fall into a panic. The one and a half hours in a borrowed Jeep take forever, and already in the admitting room of the modern St. Luke Medical Center, Christine receives an infusion. The blood count is bad, the number of platelets (thrombocytes) which are responsible for blood coagulation is far too low.

I try to hide my fear. Of course I know that everyone is praying for Christine, that everything is in God's hands, that St. Luke's is one of the best private hospitals. But I sense that Christine's will to live is ebbing. Over thirty hours of anxious waiting, the chief physician informs us that a blood transfusion would be unavoidable if the platelet count sank further. Again, unnerving waiting for the next blood test. Finally, a deep breath of relief: The count is stable. The next blood test actually shows an increase. We are incredibly relieved. Halleluja!

But Christine recovers very slowly and is further plagued by a noteworthy blow. Often she describes to me her feelings of being near death. Even after weeks of illness, her every incentive and joy regarding her gift of new life are still absent. She loses almost all of her hair and feels very weak, as if in a dark hole. Deep depression often follows in cases of severe dengue infection.

As Christine finally flies to Switzerland with the children for four weeks in order to find herself again in familiar surroundings and hopefully gather new life strength, I become thoughtful. Is it time already to take down our "tents" in the Philippines? If the situation would demand it, I am ready to do so. But so many things with Onesimo are still in a state of transition or construction, so insecure still our coworkers and services. I hope and pray that Christine will recover in Switzerland so that we can complete the pioneer phase of this work together.

But if I am honest: I, too, am tired. The last months were perhaps the most difficult of the last years. When Christine and the children return, we will have been living at the garbage dump for one year. It is time for a new, perhaps last, move. Isabel must go to school, and her Philippine private school lies closer in the direction of the city center. In a slum near there I could be helpful to Christine and Jessica by opening a life-training school for girls. Three or four girls from the trash heap long for a new beginning.

Letter from Manila

January 23, 1999. Dear Ones, we've been back in Manila already a week now. The trip went like clockwork, but was miserably long! The children coped well, only the last five hours from Malaysia to Manila, with an additional landing in Saba,

Indonesia were intolerably boring for Isabel. Luckily, Noel was asleep. I myself had to fight diarrhea and extreme fatigue. I practically did not sleep at all.

We were most sincerely welcomed in Servants house. On the first day we slept in, and the day after that we looked at a possible new shack in another slum. I was positively surprised. With renovation this will be a first-class hut. Eventually, we can even build a second story for the newly planned Girls' Center. I am very much looking forward to the new place where we can play in the nearby city park at any time.

On Friday we had a family day. Isabel was as happy as a king: sleeping in, swimming in a hotel swimming pool, seeing the Disney film "A Bug's Life" at a movie theater, and then eating an ice cream at McDonald's at the end. These are just about all the leisure-time amusements that we have here. Since the children can swim on their own, we can even read the newspaper at the pool side.

Yesterday we took a five-month-old baby from the trash heap with us for a couple of hours to give the great grandmother who is raising the orphan a brief rest. Enraptured, Isabel gave the little girl who hardly seems older than one month her bottle and played with her. Today we spoke with a social worker of a foundation which takes foundlings. After a conversation with the great grandmother, she immediately took the child with her—she had asked us to search for a place for the little one. Now we are very happy that Baby Grace has a place where she will be well provided for and taken care of.

With love, Your Christian, Christine, and Children

Moving to Philcoa

For a few days now it has clearly been hotter again. The refreshing rain torrents have not taken place. The crippling midday heat must be used for a *siesta* so that one is fit again in the cooler evening.

Christine has recovered really well. A few days ago we moved to "Philcoa," a larger slum village consisting of a couple of hundred families. We have nice neighbors. Just a short stroll away from our renovated shack, we have one of the nicest parks in Manila and an air conditioned McDonald's. We are very happy that our new residence is centrally located. In the future we will be able to spend our leisure time swimming, riding bicycles (for rent in the park), and visiting our friends.

Isabel's new school is also only twenty minutes' distance with a motorcycle taxi. "Learning Tree" is a small Philippine private school which works according to the European example of small classes, many creative stimuli, and personal guidance. Teaching takes place both in English and Tagalog. After a successful attempt with German long-distance learning, we will continue to school Isabel and later also Noel at home in German, so that they will one day be able to make the transition into the Swiss school system.

Since Christine is involved in the newly founded residential care and life-training school for girls and young women, we are trying to share the work of raising the children more equally. For the life-training school we have found an appropriate little shed in our new place of residence, where Jessica has already moved in with four girls from Payatas.

The services underway up to this point are in our coworkers' good hands and need only my guidance and coordination. In the event of meetings or emergencies, I can drive there quickly with my motorcycle. We now have four therapeutic communal living groups with self-help projects: canteen, car repair, pig farming, ceramic workshop, as well as group-leadership training, and leisure-time work with hundreds of teenagers from approximately twenty slum areas—in co-operation with local groups and communities.

I have now moved my office work to the Servants house. Correspondence, accounting, and project proposals demand more time than before. Our experienced bookkeeper, Rose Pecio-Salve, who also hails from an impoverished settlement, has managed the growing financial streams of Onesimo from its beginning, with all the necessary settlements of accounts.

Joshua and his Tondo life-training program have moved to a good house in the slum that is located on legal land. The two-story building was offered to us for purchase. Once again we wrote our friends in Switzerland and in Germany, and once again they responded quickly and generously! A large private gift especially surprised me: The father of a family in Switzerland wrote that he was in a position to buy a beautiful house for his family there. Then he decided to donate ten percent of the purchase price to our house in the Tondo slum. This crucial contribution came alongside hundreds of small donations.

Now we own our first building in the city area on legal land. That will also help us to receive an official license for our work from the Welfare Office (DSWD).

Summer Camps and "Women's Work"

From the roof of the large tent, the sound of the melancholy Filipino songs of worship reach me across the way. Again, a camp day program comes to an end in Camp Rock with a good hundred participants. It is the second of seven sequential youth camps. April's evening sun paints the bay, the water, the beach, and the palms with a golden glow. Sometimes between the songs, a spontaneous joyful cry is heard: enthusiasm for life, for God, and the camp community.

Sometimes there are also tears, as last night, when our coworker Jun spoke at the campfire about the love of the Creator for us humans. Many young people wept and brought the burdens of their life to God. The beach of Camp Rock symbolizes not only salvation for many who are stranded but also gives many young slum residents the decisive incentive no longer to flee from problems into alcohol and drugs.

John moved me most of all. Once the addicted gang leader, he has been in our community for three years. His path to healing was difficult; often he wanted to give up. And now I think about him yesterday, how he knelt down with another participant who confided in him, and wept with him. John now begins to carry others. Yet, we almost lost him a few weeks ago. He was attacked in the night by a gang on the street in front of our Center in Payatas. The attackers apparently knew him from his earlier life. Two bullets penetrated his lower thigh, a third remained stuck in his shin bone. Despite the massive injury, John could run away. He felt a super-human strength, he reported later.

In contrast, the Girls' Life-Training Community is disappointing. We were warned: It is more difficult to work with homeless and neglected girls than with boys from similar backgrounds. Of the four girls who moved in with us in February, two, Amelia and Olen, were already gone a few weeks later. "We are not yet ready for an orderly life," they wrote in a thank you letter.

Now Rachel and Venus still live with us. Rachel develops splendidly; she helps in the kitchen at the camp. Venus, in comparison, is deeply wounded and keeps us on the run almost without pause. She told us incredible stories of abuse, and since she could credibly claim that she had no parents, we took her in. Now we are clarifying whether she would be better off in a clinic.

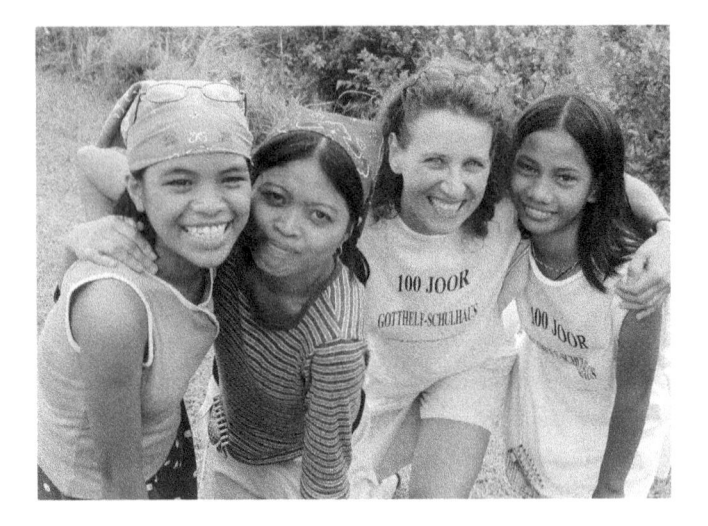

New coworkers and eleven new girls from the street and the garbage dump were a true challenge

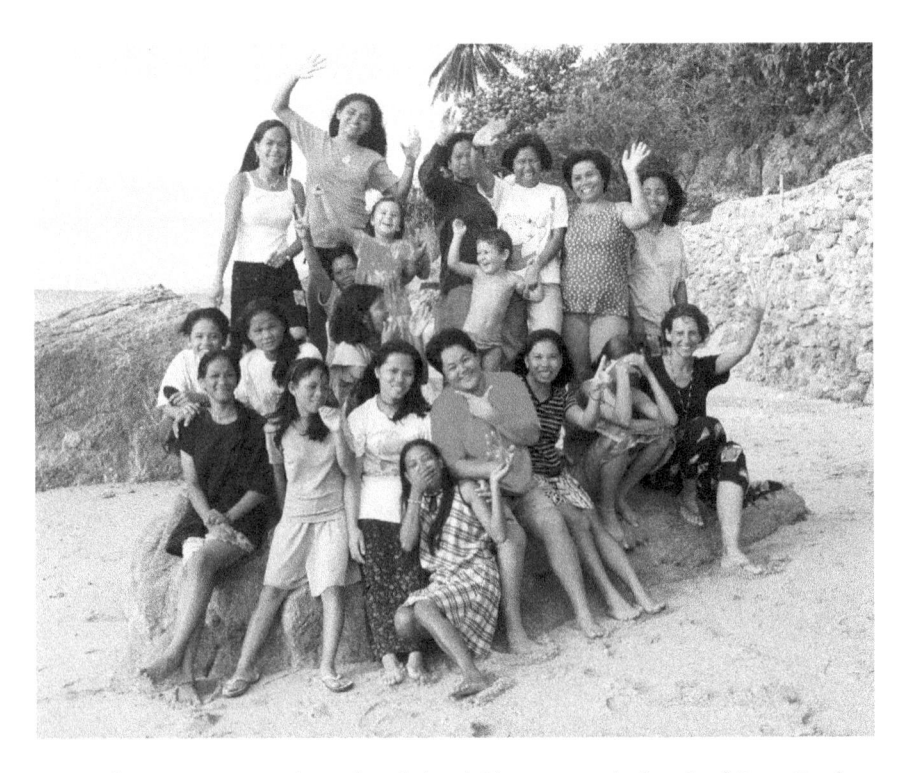

The Girls' Community with Noel, Isabel and Christine on the beach of Camp Rock. Christine's language aide, Jessica, in white T-shirt in front. Above left (with hands raised), Hazel.

The Community of Girls

It's already July. Somewhat worn out, but happily we accompanied eighteen girls and young women who had completed our first "Drug-Withdrawal Week for Girls" in Camp Rock back to Manila last evening. Christine had the primary responsibility and was experiencing high stress while I cared for children and household.

Now the pressure abates and the relief about the good outcome of the week spreads far and wide. New coworkers and eleven new contacts from the street and the garbage collection depot were a big challenge. After hesitations at the beginning, the new participants did find trust and comfort. Here, too, there were tears and shocking life stories of abuse, drugs, and violence. God's presence and healing love were palpable.

Now five of the girls are ready to join a life-training school with Onesimo. The others want to remain in contact with us. Our greater family at our new slum residence will grow to fourteen people. It is our second attempt to establish the first Onesimo Rehab Center for Girls and Young Women! Without doubt, a couple of demanding weeks lie ahead of us.

Venus will no longer be a part of it. We had to find accommodations for the eighteen-year-old in a state-sponsored home for women. She wore down our nerves incredibly, because we never knew what she would do next. She was very cunning and manipulated us all. In the three months that she lived with us as a family, we gave her countless opportunities that she did not use. We hope that Venus received so much love from us that she will never forget it. Perhaps we can dare to try again with her at a different time.

The two-week drug-withdrawal camp for boys was no less gripping. Ten new participants joined our three communities for boys, more than ten others had to be placed on a waiting list. For them, that means either back on the street or back to the rubble. That almost breaks our hearts.

At the moment I am sitting in an air conditioned hospital room at Noel's sick bed. For six days he has had a fever, has eaten almost nothing, and only taken liquids. Our good pediatrician immediately admitted him to the hospital. Noel bravely withstood blood tests, infusions, and so forth, as long as Mommy was nearby. Today, on the second day in the hospital, our three-year-old is getting better. Tomorrow or the day after we will know whether he has caught a strong influenza, typhoid, or dengue fever.

Letter from Manila

Philcoa, August 26, 1999. Last week two of the girls from the street that we took into the community flew into a rage and raved and screamed for hours, as if possessed. The trigger was a fight between the two. The other girls, and also we coworkers, were very much affected and also somewhat afraid. With prayer and much attention, the situation calmed down. We explained to the girls how they could free themselves from evil powers and extreme rage with God's help. They reconciled. At last Sunday's church service, they performed an expressive dance. I wept with joy.

Recently I bought myself fresh flowers again. Some of my neighbors and friends looked at the bouquet in astonishment, touched the flowers and said: "They are really beautiful, almost as beautiful as artificial flowers!" Yes, our cultures are opposite in so many ways. I really had to smile. But I am now slowly entering a phase, after five years in the Philippines, in which I am not entirely sure if I could and would live in Switzerland again. I have come to terms with so much here. I enjoy the positive side of life, as for example, the spontaneity. Much love, Christine

Our Neighbors, the Billionaires

The interest-free loan for the old Spaghetti House has been repaid according to its terms—thanks to the help of many friends in Switzerland and Germany. We could even enlarge Camp Rock—although its presence is a point of contention for the neighbors, since it is located in an area attractive to tourists. We sense hostilities, also on the part of the local authorities. First they prohibited us from raising tents on the beach; later they forbade campfires because the white sand would become black. Since then we light fires no less happily, but with a tin plate as a base.

During the last rain season, a heavy storm hovered over the group of islands for weeks. As a result, the steep slope behind the house became so saturated that it threatened to slide down. With much trust and little money we decided to secure the slope with deep concrete footings. At the same time we were able to create a flat parking area and a basketball court. Underneath, space for a second large house for the boys with assembly hall and toilet space was also created.

The realization of the project with the corrupt and hostile local authorities was a particular war of nerves. Time and again I traveled to the capital of the island, where the people enjoyed having me wait and then made new demands again and again. I had to demonstrate obstinacy and patience until they grasped that we were not prepared to pay bribes.

Finally, the rough brick work was finished, but money for the completion of the structure was still not in hand. There is a lot of money everywhere on this beach . . . some 800 yards distant, a family clan of Spanish descent own three beautiful beach houses. The family members spend only a few days per year here. Sometimes they fly to their property in helicopters, sometimes they come on their luxury yacht.

As a chatty neighbor, I became acquainted with the caretaker as well as the architect of these billionaires. One day the architect proudly showed me the gorgeous houses built by hand from Filipino materials. He even showed me through the beautiful living spaces. When he found out that we had run out of money to complete our Camp House, he encouraged me to ask the "Doña" (her noble Spanish title), the mother of the family, for help. She is a woman with a good heart and has always supported local projects and even founded foundations herself, he said.

With some tenacity I was successful in getting a letter of solicitation with our brochure to the personal secretary of the Doña. Her office is on the thirty-fifth floor of the most modern skyscraper in the heart of Makati, the most important commercial center of the capital city. The splendid building, in which the Philippine Stock Exchange is also housed, belongs to the family. Words almost failed me at its architectonic-beauty and its size.

Days later I called the secretary of the Doña to ask about the status of my request. "You are in luck," the lady said on the phone, "the Doña is currently spending a few days in the Philippines." I was in good humor and waited for a phone call or letter. Indeed, a letter did arrive, namely from the mayor, in which he rescinded, effective immediately, various permits and licenses for Camp Rock and the building site. The reason: A drug rehabilitation center would impede the attraction of tourists.

After the Doña read my letter, she flew to Camp Rock in her helicopter to take a look at our building site, and immediately thereafter appeared personally at the mayor's office to complain about us, because the drug addicted and street children do not belong on her beach, and because the planned new building would certainly not fit into her pretty surroundings.

I visited the mayor. Not in his government office, but rather at home. Without making an appointment. On a Sunday. With a short, fervent prayer. My mouth was dry and I could hear my heart beating in my head as I knocked on the door. A young man led me to the parlor. The mayor rose out of his chair.

His fat face with its permanent smile and mustache was only too familiar to me, not least from wall posters.

I explained to him in as friendly a manner as possible, that the entire episode was a misunderstanding: "First of all, we are not running a drug-rehab center on the beach. Secondly, in all the years that we've been there, we've not had a single drug-related incident. And thirdly, we had planned to cover the new building with Filipino materials such as bamboo and rattan anyway."

The mayor shrugged his shoulders. "The Doña is an important taxpayer here. Why did you ask her for money, anyway? For the first time, the Doña personally visited me, because of your situation!"

Depressed, I slinked back home. After some brooding and praying, the fighting spirit returned. A back-and-forth that grated on the nerves ensued, letters and faxes circulated between the mayor, the Doña, our attorney Harry Roque, and me. Lady Filthyrich actually took the opportunity to explain to us by fax from the Peninsula Hotel in New York that she was only concerned about the harmony and beauty of the area.

Harry almost exploded with rage. "Gracious me! These people have occupied our land for hundreds of years—are they still like this?"

Now Harry submitted the supporting documents and my correspondence together with an article of a well-known journalist to the national television station and to the largest daily newspaper in the Philippines. Harry is also the chief of staff of a well-known parliamentarian in Manila who, I found out, would soon have a conversation with the governor of the island, who would put in a good word with our mayor on our behalf.

When two weeks had passed and nothing had happened, I visited the mayor yet another time, again at his home. I was nervous and the atmosphere was tense, but I tried to remain as objective as possible. As an aside, I inserted into the conversation the fact that the story of "the surprising conclusion" was now at the television station and with the editors of the newspaper.

The mayor's blood shot to his face and he screamed at me, "What, you want to threaten me!" As calmly as possible, I replied: "What other option do we little people have against such a powerful family?" Enraged, I was sent away.

The work at the building site of Camp Rock stood still. More days elapsed. Then finally an answer came from the office of the mayor in the form of an agreement which we were to sign if we wanted to reinstate the permit for Camp Rock and the building site. The agreement consisted of a list of demands in which we found nothing that we didn't want anyway. But with our acquiescence, the Doña and the authorities could at least somewhat save face.

The means for the completion of Camp Rock actually came together in time, as always. Our co-fighters in Europe don't have billions, but they are wonderful, noble, and loyal!

Trust is Priceless

It's impossible that it's already June 2000. So much has happened since last fall. Our fifty fosterlings survived Christmas and New Year's well. On January 22, we celebrated in the open the eighteen teenagers who completed the first six months in the new community. It is incredible to experience how young people can change in a half year, when they are loved and cared for.

From March until May we were in Switzerland on our second home vacation, if one can call it a "vacation. " In any case, a tour with forty events was a part of it. We reported to church congregations, home circles, schools, youth groups. It touched us to see how many friends stand behind us and carry us. No wonder that we have experienced so many blessings and successes in the last years. The children enjoyed the many playgrounds, bicycling, and their cousins. Nonetheless, after just a few days, Noel wanted to go "home to Manila" again.

During our stay in Switzerland, a new leisure-time series took place in Camp Rock, this time with "only" 450 participants. Shortly before the series, an old, worn-out ferry sank on the crossing to our vacation island, and many people died. Frightened by this occurrence, some who had signed up decided against coming. The eighty young coworkers from various slums and their base communities, who were trained by our team before the start of the New Year, appear to have conducted themselves well in the camps.

We had already decided last fall to leave the work of Onesimo to the Filipinos in three years, and to return to Switzerland for good. Isabel will then be nine-years-old and can spend her important teenage years in Switzerland. This time table is also helpful to us in the difficult-to-bear moments in the slum.

On the day after our return, as we stood waiting for thirty minutes for a taxi at the edge of the street, with our children and some baggage, dripping with sweat and enveloped by exhaust fumes, I noticed tears in Christine's eyes. Before we went to sleep, she read the solution to me, Psalm 20:2: "The Lord hears you in your misery!" She said: "We need that again now, don't we." And then we prayed together.

A nice surprise on Sunday morning was a visit from Venus and John. On the advice of our psychiatrist, we had brought Venus to a women's facility last year, from which she ran away a short time later. John again brought her to us after that and explained that he loved her and would marry her. And now they were here . . . with their baby.

As before, Venus needs constant attendance, complains about annoyances, hears imaginary voices, and refuses medication. I asked John how he manages to cope with Venus. "It is difficult, but I love Venus," he replies.

"And how is it going with your work?" I ask him. John works as messenger for Harry's legal practice in the commercial district of Makati.

He said: "It's going super. I'm treated well. At the beginning I had to pick up a large amount of money. They asked me if I would run away with the money. I replied: 'Don't be afraid—I can always get money somewhere; trust, on the other hand, is priceless.'"

Letters from Manila

Philcoa, in June 2000. We've been back in Manila for a week now. Our neighbors greeted us affectionately: "Good to have you back. You've gotten quite fat, haven't you . . ." Already after a day or two, Switzerland is far away for me—too bad! And we're packing and unpacking again! I have the feeling as if my entire life consists of packing and traveling. In the first couple of days here I would have liked to take a plane back to Switzerland.

The tin roof of our shack is not leak proof. While we were in Switzerland, the children in the neighborhood apparently used the roof as a playground. Our helpful neighbor, "Boy," has taken on the repairs in exchange for daily wages. While he and his friends replace pieces of tin with holes in them, a gale-force rain shower surprises us. Now water pours in everywhere, on the sofa, the beds, the floor. . . . I quickly place containers around, but the water is faster, puddles are beginning to form. Then I smell smoke and notice that the rainwater drips directly into a wall socket. It sparks and smokes, and in my mind I already see our hut in flames. With racing heart, I run to the fuse box. Just in time!

Boy comes again the next day. He is supposed to glue synthetic tiles onto our cement floor so that it will be easier to keep clean. We move our few pieces of furniture into the corner and head to work and to school.

When I return home in the afternoon, I think I'm going to have a stroke: The entire interior of the shack, my only private sphere, is covered in a thick red layer of dust. In order to even out the red cement floor, Boy had to use a sanding machine. The children, who arrived home with Jessica a short time before me, avidly help Boy with the gluing of the tiles—in their lovely, clean clothes, of course. Then I remember that the water tank is empty, and I will have to clean without water.... That does it! I gather my last strength together, pack a few things into a bag and go to the Servants house with the children.

Chris and our house parents Margrit and David immediately see that I'm not doing well. I catch my breath, tell the story, take a shower. Spontaneously we decide to take care of correspondence and telephone calls and to reserve a room in a simple hotel tomorrow. Chris postpones several appointments until next week, Margrit and Dave bid us farewell with a gift basket full of snacks and a bouquet of roses. They, too, are glad that we are allowing ourselves this necessary break. In the hotel, we finish all the thank you notes and letters and rest at the pool. The children almost get webbed feet from so much swimming.

It takes so little in this crazy city with its constant stress to bring me to my limit. And yet—what is my stress in comparison to the fight to survive that the poor endure? Hunger, violence, fire, typhoons, relocation, catastrophes, deaths of family members, degrading situations, discrimination—most of our friends have experienced more than one of these fates. Experts say that a number of unprocessed traumas transport a person into a state of a kind of long-lasting shock. The effect is indifference, dulling of feelings, and apathy. That may well be the reason why our friends don't grasp certain opportunities: because they are missing the emotional strength to take a risk. Many young people are accustomed to taking the path of least resistance. They live only in the moment and simply give in to their moods and feelings. Only when they have learned to persevere and maintain do they have the possibility of finding a good job.

Our beloved Mylene, who now has been with us and belongs to Onesimo for a year (and who had to process more than what Arol did to her), has just run away for a second time. On the way to school, the now thirteen-year-old ran into her old gang friends and her "boyfriend." Because of a momentary desire for physical love and recognition, she threw all our care, the new school, and the security of the Girls' Center overboard in order to get what she thought she needed at the moment. We are sad that this dear girl and the beloved friend of both our children has given up. At the same time, we know that our help is a voluntary offer. We strongly hope that Mylene will come back of her own accord.

This week Venus and her sweet baby are living with us. John desperately needs a break from her! Already after a few days we could fill half of a book with crazy stories. But she has also taken small steps forward. Until now she had a panicked fear of water and showered rarely. She also never wanted to wash dishes.

Yesterday I almost had to force her to take a shower. It was urgently necessary! I went with her into our tiny toilet, in which one also showers. We made the water extra warm so that it would be pleasant. I prayed with her and encouraged her. As I poured the warm water over her with the beaker, she screamed as if impaled on a spike: "Please, Christine, don't kill me!" Fortunately it was raining heavily outside at the time. I hoped that there would not be a gathering crowd in response to the cries for help.

Payatas in the World News

July 10, 2000, Monday morning, about 8:00 o'clock. Unsuspecting, I turn into the street that leads to our Center for Boys and to the dump site. Something isn't quite right. Hundreds of people are running in the direction of a smokestack. My heart begins hammering, and I begin running.

Minutes later I am horrified: Where there were many shacks still standing yesterday, lies a considerably higher "avalanche cone" of wet, decaying garbage. After two weeks of hurricane-like rains, the ninety-foot high and mile-long mountain of rubbish slid into the slum below.

At the edge, flattened shacks are in flames. The fire crackles, people scream, a Jeepney full of children, some badly burned, races away. The nearest hospital is at least an hour distant! A chain of people forms around the burning huts; making a panicked effort, they pass water buckets to one another—which, in light of the wind-stoked fire, is a hopeless endeavor. Mothers scream for their children, who have disappeared; children cry for their mothers.

A despairing teenager tries, with bare hands, to dig his father out of the rubble. The approximately forty-year-old man lies trapped up to his belt under tin roof, wooden posts, and garbage. He's having trouble breathing: "I can't make it, hurry, hurry . . ."

"Where is Mother?" wails the son.

"She went to work; keep it up, hurry . . ." the father wheezes. We grab like crazy, but the wet garbage is heavy and compact, almost like stone. There are too few to help! They are afraid, and I understand why: Shacks are breaking apart, downed cables are lying around, and at any moment, more garbage can begin to slide. It is a haunting scene.

Someone hands me a crowbar; someone else comes with a lifting jack. Now it's going forward: I arrange for water, which the unlucky stranger gratefully slurps out of a plastic lid. Suddenly, enough helpers are there, and I slink away—I have to get to the Onesimo center.

I rarely cover the 200 yards to our residential community as quickly as today. Then a stone falls from my heart: The boys from our Center were spared. Even two of them who were on the mountain gathering leftovers for the pigs managed to escape with only a great fright.

Twenty-four hours later I experience something that I never had before, in all my years in the slum: The world comes calling. Live cameras everywhere, international television and radio stations have built emergency broadcast installations and report from the horror. And when the cameras run, they are here: government representatives, government advisers, police spokesmen, many, many onlookers . . . and, of course, President Joseph Estrada, previously an actor. He, who grew up in Tondo and starred in over one hundred films—often as the avenger of the downtrodden—he, too, wants to show the world his deep empathy and demonstrate in front of the cameras how deeply concerned he is about the scavengers. Hundreds of soldiers and policemen are here, searching with sanitary masks and shovels, excavating for corpses. Yes, yes, they're doing something. Our rubbish mountain has become an event!

Ten days later they have dug out over 200 corpses, and the search continues. Health organizations still deliver trucks full of food. People literally plunge into them. We wait until the famous helpers pull out and we, with a few other local groups, and the victims remain behind.

Of course, the dump site is now closed. It could be that in a half year some journalists may come by again—and they shouldn't report then that nothing had changed!

The scavengers were offered no alternatives, however. The closing brings unemployment, hunger, and despair to thousands of people. The greatest part of the poor of this city is not registered anywhere, many don't exist statistically. They represent nothing more than an embarrassment about which one prefers not even to think. Except for elections. Then suddenly they all receive a voting voucher and an access street is paved—unavoidable, with the street sign bearing the name of the beneficent politician.

When I am quiet sometimes and all alone with myself (which happens very seldom), the horrible pictures of this misfortune go through my mind. I hear the despairing screams and the crackling fire. Then I sense that my breath is coming faster, and I think: Nothing will be as before.

Why particularly the poor? What does that mean, God? With Onesimo we fight for each individual life, and then the mountain of rubbish begins to slide and with one stroke hundreds are dead and thousands are left in even greater need, injured inside and out. It can't have been God, no. But I stand here without an answer and sometimes also enraged.

I have to call the God I know into my consciousness again and again, have to concentrate on what he says: "I was naked and sick and hungry . . ." God places himself on the side of the victims, he suffers with the deformed and injured. Why do I want to make him responsible for this happening! I want to hold fast to the thought that at the end of time he will establish his Kingdom of peace and bring everything into balance. Only in the belief in such promises can I attain inner peace. What remains is faith.

Flowing (Waste) Water

The heavy rain has stopped. But two weeks ago, it caught us too, although far more harmlessly. I brought Christine to the airport. Her grandmother in Switzerland had a heart attack with complications, and thanks to travel trip insurance, Christine could fly there for a few days. On this day it rained buckets full; as I went to bed, it was still rattling against the roof. At about 2:00 a.m., my upset neighbors literally pulled me out of bed. I didn't hear their shouts and knocking on the door, but fortunately they have a key to our home.

I slipped out of bed somewhat confused and suddenly awakened with a start. There I stood with bare feet in approximately eight inches of a filthy sauce. The wastewater canal had flowed through our shack! And the "sauce" was rising!

In feverish haste the neighbors helped me tie our mattresses under the roof with ropes. I packed shoes, books, laundry, papers and other things that weren't wet yet into plastic bags and nailed them as high as possible on the posts and plywood walls. Then there was enough time to wake Noel and Isabel, before they got wet. The three of us retreated to the last dry spot in our little house, the upper story of the children's bunk beds. From there we observed how the dirty water level almost reached table-surface height. With my cell phone, I called the Girls' Center and the Frisco community, which also lie along a river. They were safe in the upper story of their houses, I was told. The water was high, but everything was under control and everyone in good humor...

I was glad that Christine didn't have to experience this. She presumably was sitting comfortably in a jet high above in the sky, somewhere between Manila and Zurich. Unlike me, she becomes very attached to places and residences. This would have affected her very deeply. For Isabel and Noel it was above all an adventure.

The "sauce" climbed higher and higher. At some point it became too dangerous and unpleasant for me—the three of us on the bed over the moving water. I grabbed Isabel and Noel each under an arm and waded with them out into the night in front of laughing neighbors. Filipinos like to laugh—and often, it is their way to process something emotional. We went to a higher-lying part of our neighborhood, where I could leave my two little ones on dry ground for the rest of the night.

The river receded almost as quickly as it had risen. An evil smelling, sticky slime that covered everything was left behind. Schools were closed because many streets in Manila were flooded. Our boys from Payatas were already standing in front of the door in the early morning and helped with all aspects of the clean-up. Their house near the mountain of rubble was spared from the high water.

We had to throw some things away immediately. We tried saving some letters, photos, and a few books and magazines with a hairdryer and with the help of the sun. Our children were particularly sad about the loss of their guinea pigs. In the night, instead of the little animals in their box on the floor, the father thought about the expensive sewing machine....

Controversy about Corpses

Since the rubble slide in July, that is, a good four months ago, I have been at the edge of its "mass grave" a couple of times and have wept with the survivors. Once I witnessed these terrible scenes: Soldiers placed the crushed and deformed remains of human bodies next to one another on the ground of the village plaza, so that survivors could identify them. Most of the facial features were difficult to recognize or not at all. I saw how men and women fought about the corpses. Each wanted at least to say goodbye to their child, their brother and sister, mother or father. And the government had promised affected families a sum of money for each deceased family member.

Misery and hunger on the trash heap are more brutal than before. The mountain stands still, the work is gone, and for scavengers there is no state-supported public welfare. The search for additional victims was discontinued in the meantime. Until now 234 corpses were identified; seventy-three families were still missing members. Lived on the trash; died under the trash.

Last week families demonstrated in a sit-down strike in front of the city administration building. They demanded, finally, the payment of the 15,000 *pesos* in "emergency relief," promised by the government representatives in the first hours in front of the cameras. Further, they demanded the handing over of the remains of fifty deceased, who had been held back for months "for exact identification." The approximately fifty courageous strikers were driven away by a hundred-strong contingent of police and strike-breaking forces, but managed nonetheless to attain a hearing with the city president. He promised again the distribution of the support monies mentioned. He also would immediately order the continuing search for the remaining victims in the rubble.

Beautiful words. The media was present.

Of the survivors, many moved away or were "relocated." A large part of the remaining slum residents have no work any longer and therefore more hunger. Private assistance organizations distribute food to hundreds of them every day. We are glad that we can at least give our approximately twenty youngsters from Payatas a home in our communities. Jun Arizala, our leader of the Onesimo community in Payatas, is actually fully in charge of the care and control of our boys. Despite that, in the time of need he had agreed to contribute even more fully: as president of a neighborhood organization in Payatas. Those landowners adjacent to our slum wanted to use the time of confusion to their benefit and tried to close the access street to the settlements of the poor with a large fence. Thanks to Jun's intervention, the local authorities were able to hinder the erection of this fence.

Everything that we do here is sensitive . . .

Joachim and Sieglinde Hammer have checked in at the Manila International Airport. Tomorrow is New Year's Eve, and they will again be back in OJC Reichelsheim. We had just been sharing exciting days in Camp Rock, preparing for the summer camps in 2001 and training teenagers to be small-group leaders. Joachim truly bubbled over with enthusiasm about the creative and experience-oriented Bible-discussion circles in the Camp.

On the way home from the airport, my cell phone rings: Randy, our youngest garbage picker and glue sniffer from Payatas is lying in the emergency room of the government hospital in the provincial city of Batangas. On the trip to Camp Rock, the ferry's loading ramp, weighing tons, had squashed his foot.

Two hours later I stand in the hospital, a single story flat building that is hardly trust inspiring. Randy's foot looks bad. Nevertheless, I still clearly recognize three whole toes in the bloody mass. I introduce myself as a medical care professional and Randy's care provider and ask about the procedure.

"Amputation, Sir," the physician replies drily—simple injury delimitation, third world medicine, not more. One must avoid a life-threatening infection and as soon as possible, the doctor explains. Don't they have a surgeon who could sew the foot back together, I ask. "Such serious injuries are handled only by amputation here in the city."

"Then Randy must be taken to Manila, and quickly!" I declare, very emphatically. The physician ponders only a moment. "Good, if you want to risk such a transport then I will provide an ambulance for you. But I can't delegate a doctor to accompany—the responsibility is yours."

The trip is fretful. Sometimes we proceed with open roads and loud sirens, but all too often we crawl in mile-long traffic jams, against which even flashing lights and sirens are powerless. And as we turn on the radio and hear the breaking news, another hammer blow: A series of bomb attacks in the capital with a number of fatalities and hundreds of injured. Of all times!

After almost three hours we are in greater Manila. The streets are perfect chaos, but at least the police escort us with flashing lights to the Orthopedic Center. There I almost have a stroke: Examination rooms and corridors are completely crowded, like a military hospital in the war after a battle. On improvised bedsteads and cots the injured lie, moaning. In a semi-dark corner I see a young woman, motionless. One of her legs is torn off at the thigh, the stump is tied on with a rubber tube, the bandage saturated with blood. Apparently she is waiting for an available surgeon.

A stressed nurse informs us that in the afternoon within an hour five bombs exploded, one at the airport, another in an overcrowded overhead railway just by the hospital.

"We can save the foot," a doctor says, "but the young man has to wait a while." The little while lasted seven hours. Unbelievably long hours. The operation then was successful, according to information from the surgeon. If the foot heals without complications, Randy can learn to walk again in the coming months.

In the following days, the media reported twenty-two dead and hundreds of injured. President Estrada exhorted the population to remain calm. Naturally, he is nervous, since proceedings to effect his removal from office are being brought because of accusations of corruptibility. Perpetrators of the attack were the Islamic group Abu Sayyaf.

Exactly fifteen days later it has come to this: A half-million Filipinos drive President Joseph Estrada out of the government palace. Hours later Vice President Gloria Arroyo is sworn in. We are very happy about the victory of the non-violent peoples' uprising, but our gratitude and our tears of joy on this historic day are also for the seventeen young people who have completed the first six months of their rehabilitation. At the concluding celebration in front of 150 relatives and friends from the slums they report that with help from Christ they are on their way to a life with direction and dignity. That is the true revolution!

Nevertheless, the longer we do this the more I have the feeling that it simply isn't enough. It's not enough to enable the poor—with some guidance, a good economic self-help project and the discovery of a living personal faith—to stand up and help themselves. They need their share of the goods of this world. Justice. And we rich would do good to share our good fortune with the economically disadvantaged, before we perish from obesity, heart attacks, environmental neglect, or by terrorism, which is also a result of this imbalance.

Poor and rich, north and south need each other. Both must seek a common understanding that God loves all people the same. Together we can empower each other significantly.

In two years, for the good of our children, we will finally return to Switzerland. Until then we should work to develop a loving partnership between the people in Europe and those here in the slums. A thought comes to me: How would it be if on our last vacation at home in a few weeks, we would take along two or three of our young people? Our friends in Europe would suddenly see the faces, hear the voices, live, and not through the "Schneider filter."

Logically, this is potentially sensitive in execution. But everything that we do here is delicate. Those who only do what is not sensitive, do nothing.

Three Filipinos in Switzerland

June 12, 2001. Once again, we're sitting in an airplane, flying in the direction of Manila. The six weeks in Switzerland were no vacation, but rather a marathon of events. Next to me sits Jose (25), formerly a boy of the streets and nightclub dancer. Next to him is Allen, the leader of a scavenger gang, of which most members entered our second rehab program, and in the back is Gerald, the former thief and pimp. When I think how Dr. Randy advised us at that time to turn Gerald immediately out into the street, that he was psychotic, he heard voices, and was a danger to all of us ... and when I think how he and the two others have described their lives to our friends for weeks now, almost every evening. No question. There sit three miracles! I am glad that our coworkers chose Jose, Allen, and Gerald to make the trip.

Naturally they were stopped by the police at the airport in Zurich. "They didn't like our faces," Jose said afterwards, but Allen found that it was not out of order on their part. "The police treated us with respect, not like in Manila."

I was especially moved when Gerald told a group of young Swiss teenagers that he didn't envy them for their possessions or their beautiful country, but because they were able to grow up in a family in which they were considered worthwhile, and were raised with love and discipline. That's what he had always wished for. The reactions of the young people were incredible. One visitor got right to the point: "It was for me as if all cultural and material barriers and differences were overcome."

Perhaps thanks to Onesimo, lasting relationships between people in Europe and in the slums will grow. Now they're not simply "the poor," they are brothers and sisters with faces. Three such faces have now been seen by our friends in Switzerland and Germany.

September 11th

Two weeks have now gone by since September 11, 2001. For two weeks there have been no other stories in the media on any other subject. An incomprehensible day with an incomprehensible event: On this September 11, 2001, 35,615 children world wide died of malnutrition, just as every day, according to a world nutrition organization.

Letter from Manila

Manila, October 11, 2001. My Dear Ones, our new residence, our fifth slum house to date, is splendid. It is an old tin shack, and it stands almost in the middle of the last rice fields of Manila, population 14 million. We are happy about our own little garden and running water—which, of course, must be filtered.

In the evening as we fall asleep, we don't hear any drunken neighbors yelling, but rather the chirping of crickets and the croaking of frogs. Often I lie down with a feeling of true good fortune and enjoy the quiet! Far away in the distance, the traffic drones on without letup. And because our new shack is located only two-hundred yards from our old settlement, our children haven't lost their friends. On the contrary, they are happy about our small courtyard for playing.

From 7:00 a.m. until noon, Isabel and Noel are in school. That means a lot of free time for me for housework, planting flowers, and so forth. On two afternoons during the week, Christian takes care of the children, and I work in the office. The weekends in the last few months are mostly unplanned and true family days. This is really a new development in the Schneider family.

Furthermore, three days ago we acquired household help for our little residence. This is how it happened: Just by chance, I overhear the ten-year-old neighbor boy Bongbong speaking to Noel: "Tomorrow Macmac and I will be taken to our relatives in the provinces. I won't see you for a long time, maybe one or two Christmases from now, and not on your birthday either." Noel is upset. I also get involved in the conversation and pose a few questions. I have a sense of foreboding.

Subsequently I pay Bongbong's mother a visit in her tiny house on the foul-smelling wastewater canal. Marie-Jane tells me that she found out a few months ago that for four years, her husband has had a second wife and family. Her husband has no legal responsibilities as pertains to her because they, as most of the slum couples, are not legally married. When he comes to visit he treats Marie-Jane as his wife, of course, who stands at his disposal. That is part of her "service," since he still takes care of his children to a degree. Sometimes he brings something to eat. Marie-Jane wants him to leave her alone, however. That means that she would get no money from him whatsoever. She would have to watch her children go hungry and no longer attend school.

Now she plans to take the boys to the husband's relatives in the provinces. "What else can I do?" she complains to me, crying. "There my sons at least will get something to eat. And hopefully my husband won't come for any more visits."

I know only too well from our Onesimo charges that children staying with relatives without their parents are often terribly neglected. Many had to work as house slaves and suffered blows and even torture daily. Without someone who stands by them, they are lost. I tell Marie-Jane all this so that she can think it over: "You know, your children need their mother's love perhaps even more than food. Although food is urgently necessary too, I know."

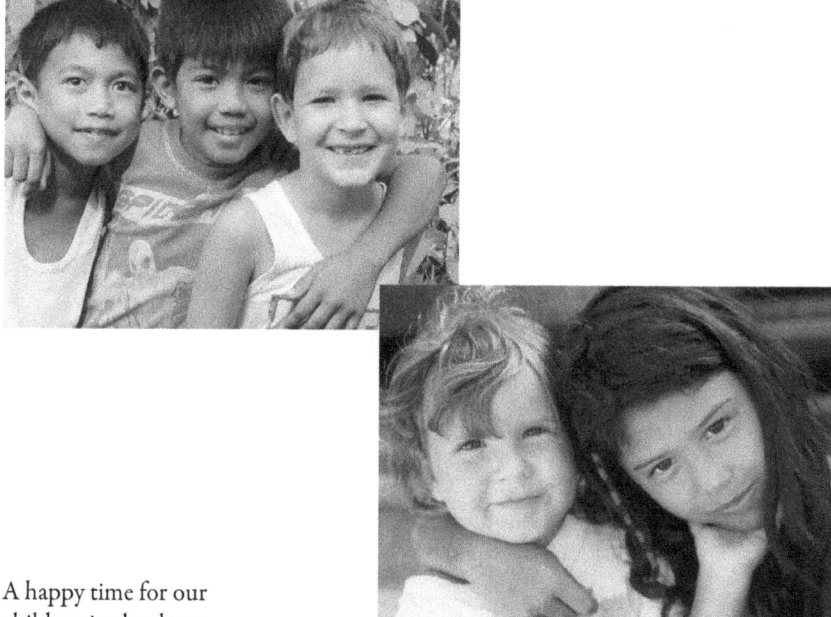

A happy time for our children in the slums

And so, Christian and I talk that same evening about a possible solution. We know many, many mothers in the adjacent neighborhood who are overtaxed. But these two boys play in our house every day and almost belong to the family. Their sad eyes, which mirror bad premonitions, break my heart.

And so it comes to pass that three days ago, Marie-Jane came to cook for us. She helps me with my housework, and I can leave her alone with all of the children from time to time. As a result, I can write, go shopping, or even spend a free evening with Christian. In the evenings I am tired from the ups and downs of the day, but very happy. From time to time, Bongbong and Macmac present me with a smile. What a reward for being willing to share a little of our private sphere. Over the weekends, we'll continue to be together as a family. Marie-Jane will be able to make do with her small weekly wages.

Next Wednesday we will receive exalted visitors in our shack: The Swiss ambassador and his deputy want to see how we can live in the slum. They read a story about us in Schweizer Familie *[Swiss Family magazine]. I will make sure that they also take a glance at the tiny hut on the wastewater canal, in which one of the real heroines lives.*

Much love, Christine

A Bridge between Rich and Poor

Recently I have become the proud owner of a dagger. The eighteen-year-old Jun-Jun asked me for 50 *pesos*. He has gambling debts, he begged, and if he can't pay them, something bad will happen. I shook my head, although I noticed the fear in his eyes and in his voice. But we don't ever give any cash, he knows that.

Finally, Jun-Jun says: "If you don't help me, I'll have to rob someone; you don't give me any choice."

"You are much too smart to commit such a stupid act," I reply.

Then he pulled an approximately sixteen-inch-long dagger out of his shorts and screamed at me: "You don't believe me? I will do it!"

"I'll buy the dagger from you, for 50 *pesos*," I say. He ponders for a short moment and nods. A handshake and the deal was done. Since then I am the owner of a dagger; who would believe *that*?

In the meantime, we're already writing the year 2002, the seventh year of Onesimo. At this point, all the camps, the school/training programs, all regularly scheduled events are being organized and presented by the Filipinos. We Schneiders are, above all, friends and mentors to these mostly young coworkers. And naturally we are still active as important fundraisers.

More than eighty people now live and work with Onesimo. Most importantly, it is our faithful friends in Europe who finance the work through contributions or sponsorships.

This sounds normal, but this "business plan" doesn't satisfy me. At the beginning we believed that we would be able to establish a profit-making business project that would allow our quickly growing social work to stand on its own financial feet. But we were naïvely idealistic. We underestimated the murderous economic competition, the inhuman demands of the work, and the corruption. Short and sour: Onesimo is still surviving on donations from Europe.

My expectations of the "rich" and of the Christian churches here in Manila were also naïve. When I think back on all my unsuccessful attempts at contact in the last few years...

Once we were invited by the foundation of a thriving bank. Beforehand, in preparation they demanded a written description of an appropriate project proposal. We had a fine meal in the stylish penthouse of the bank's skyscraper, followed by a photo shoot, at which the Director handed us a check for the equivalent of 500 US dollars.... We were cleverly misused for the bank's public relations.

In large, with well-to-do churches it was often similar: empty promises and commiserations. I was always careful not to approach churches that already supported a street-children initiative.

I attended religious services, alone or with the team, often in air conditioned churches with carpets and terrific sound systems for the worshipful devotional music. And then the services were in English instead of Tagalog, so that my poor friends could understand very little. Sometimes I was actually glad that they couldn't, such as the time when an apparently prominent woman told of God's saving her in a business crisis, in which she lost absolutely everything: "*I went down to only one car...*" For her, the ownership of a single car meant that she had lost "absolutely everything," and she wept as she spoke! Good that my friends from the slum didn't understand most of what she said.

I think about Conny, the theologian who was writing her doctoral dissertation and suddenly appeared to lecture me avidly about the fact that the residents of the slums would have been better off to stay in their provinces, where they would do better, and one should work to return them to their original homes. This is basically true, and I asked her where she had come from. The province of Bicol, she replied, fourteen hours south of Manila. There her family owns a large house with land. I kept hammering away to determine why she had come to Manila. Her answer was, "Our children need a good education, and they can get one only in the capital city."

As if the poor didn't have even more right to seek a future for their children in the city, to seek work, food, and an improvement of the circumstances of their lives.

Again and again, I hear these stereotypical answers and prejudgments about the poor: Many don't have to live in the slums, but do so because it's so much more comfortable for them. Most of them are hiding there because they are lazy or they are criminals. With this logic, approximately four million people are lazy or criminals, the majority of whom are children!

Repeatedly, wealthy Christians told me this, and added that most of them are professional slumlords—that is, people who build additional houses in the slums and rent them to poor families. But in my experience, these slumlords represent perhaps ten percent of the slum population. And often they play the role of vital entrepreneur, organizing support from the public assistance offices which may provide water and power or relief in times of fire and flood.

Naturally there were also splendid encounters in fundraising. There is the owner of a well-known private Swiss bank whom I was permitted to visit in his office in Zurich, who doubles the donations that come from Philippine contributors every year—and who absolutely wants to remain anonymous. There is the Swiss with a Philippine passport, a director of a famous pharmaceutical firm, who generously supports Onesimo to this day, out of his own pocket. There is the Union Church of Makati in the middle of the commercial district of Manila, which substantially supports various projects for the poor. And, despite everything, there are again and again among the educated Filipino population, Christians who forego well paid careers in the free market or in another country and who engage in relief work or NGOs with comparatively low salaries. And that, while 14,000 trained health care professionals leave the Philippines each year in order to earn good salaries outside the country, and on top of that each year 5,000 Filipino physicians re-train to get licenses as healthcare professionals in other countries so that they can pursue their fortune.

We urgently need a bridge between the poor and the rich in Manila, and a bridge between the wealthy North and West and the poor South and East.

Letters from Manila

March 2002. We Schneiders have now been living in the Philcoa slum for over three years. We never before as a family lived in the same place for such a long time. Again and again during this time, I have longed to read the Bible and have discussions with my neighbors and friends from the settlement. But deep within me, something prevented me from approaching them. I limited myself to being a neighbor and friend, to share our lives, to admit limitations and weaknesses, to accept and give help, and to seek peace after an argument. And then, after almost exactly three years, my neighbor and friend Shine asks me through a third person if we could read the Bible together. Wow!

Now we meet each week in her shack to read the Gospel of Matthew while other neighbors pursue their own leisure activity, gambling. Because of her own life full of deprivation and suffering, Shine understands the Bible texts often at the first attempt. She feels close to the simple life of Jesus and his followers. Often I listen to her, spellbound, as she speaks about her new experiences with God: answering prayers, when her three children are ill; difficulty, when her husband is almost stabbed in front of their shack; consolation, when the money isn't enough for food and school; reconciliation, with the long-estranged neighbor.

A few women have jokingly named Shine "the saint" because of our meetings. But a week ago, two new women joined us to read the Bible: for one, Marie-Jane, who lives with us half-days with her three children, and another, Lane, whose husband is on death's row in prison because he raped her nine-year-old daughter. And now, Shine, Marie-Jane, and Lane meet each week—even when I'm not there!

Shine beams with enthusiasm about the new development. I do too. Her new faith will enlarge her horizon in the neighborhood, of that I am sure.

Philcoa, May 8, 2002. *In a few days we leave again for a family vacation: to Boracay, the dreamy island with white sand and tall palm trees. Unfortunately, in the meantime it has become greatly exploited as a result of the tourist trade. At the end of the high season algae grow in the shallow seawater, the paths are trampled. We'll see if it's still beautiful nonetheless.*

Our assignments at Onesimo have changed. While Chris can delegate much to his Filipino coworkers and the new leadership team, so that he sometimes feels "useless," I, after all these years in the background, am in my element. The children are becoming more independent, and therefore I have more possibilities to participate. For example, I accompany young women or even new Servants as a mentor. I find this very fulfilling. What I do is valued; nonetheless, I am free to determine how much time I will invest.

At the same time I am also happily anticipating our return to Switzerland. But I pull myself together and don't demonstrate it too overtly since I know that Chris feels completely different—perhaps as I felt then, as we left for the Philippines. Although I have become accustomed to so much, there is still a great deal here that I don't understand.

At about 5:00 p.m., when it gets a little cooler, we—as a family—often go to a beautiful park with trees and benches very near to the university. We take a blanket and picnic with us and Noel brings his bow and arrows from the mountains. Chris runs a couple of rounds, flies kites with the children, I read a book or chat with the occasional companion. Not far away there is a café with a fine chocolate cake and cold ice tea in large cups. The only thing that bothers me: We always have to undertake an act of trash collecting because the lawn is cluttered with it.

Cordial Greetings, Christine

Melancholy Christmas

Christmas will soon be here. The year 2002 comes to an end, and our time in Manila too. I would dearly love to make time stand still. My ties to this country and its people are deep.

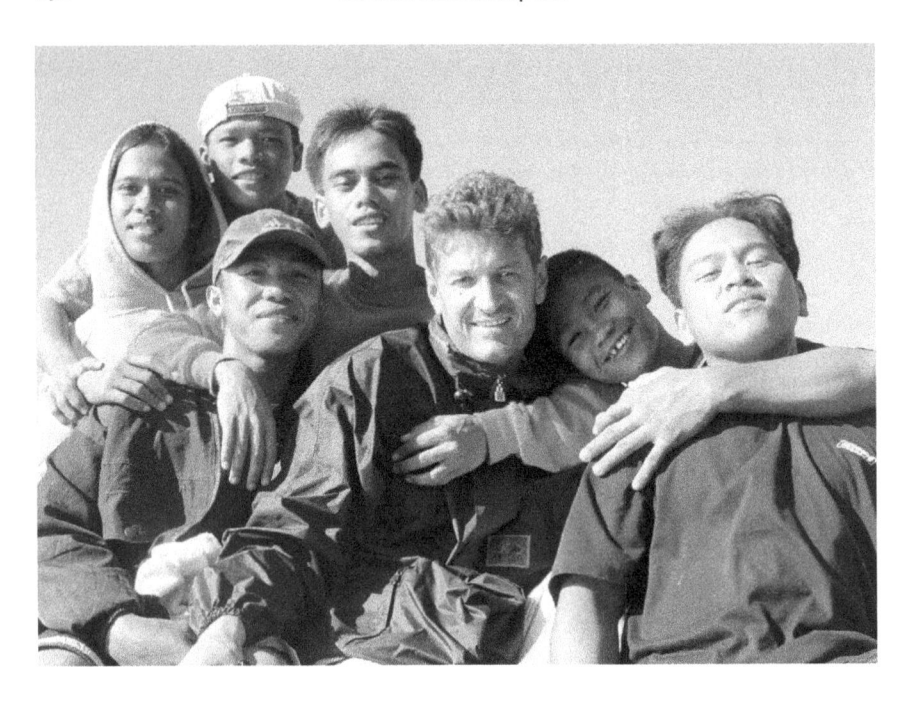

To open the eyes of young people, who literally come out of the rubble, to the wonders of nature—what could be better?

Here I experienced catastrophes of all kinds: floods, earthquakes, a volcano eruption, a rubble slide, cyclones, firestorms, revolutions, murder, and manslaughter. Here my love for Christine has deepened through joy and peril. Here in the slums our Noel was born. Here our two children have grown happily and in good health to this day and kept us fit. Here I experienced the unrestrained love of life of people who have practically nothing. Here I watched more or less helpless, as children, and young and old people, died because of hunger, illness, and violence. Here I encountered my shadow, my personal failures. Here I learned a different kind of weeping, praying, and laughing. Here I experienced hundreds of young people who conceived of a trust in God and followed a new path, as they broadened their horizons in a movement that graduated from my influence some time ago.

Three weeks ago I was able to go mountain climbing again for a few days with forty boys on a beautiful island. To open the eyes of young people who have literally come from the rubble to the wonders of nature—what could be better?

Only those that were fit were allowed to come along this time. I didn't know the area, there were no trail maps, and there was also a shortage of wind jackets and walking shoes. Just before reaching the peak, at about 4,000 feet, we were surprised by strong wind gusts and thick fog which threatened to quickly chill us. Without having reached the highest point, we began the descent to warmer regions. No one seemed disappointed. Ultimately, we had climbed so high that we stood in the middle of an actual cloud!

Most of them wore the usual flip-flops. Ariel was actually barefoot on the way, although without my knowledge: Shortly before the steep climb through the rain forest, we stopped in a village to fill our water containers and to rid ourselves of unnecessary ballast. Apparently Ariel included his flip-flops in this category. During the descent, he had to clench his teeth mightily because of his injured feet.

It took two days to get home. The hardest for me were the five hours in the Jeepney: Forty-three boys rode in this vehicle with bad suspension, which was intended for only twenty passengers, jolting over dusty natural paths and through little rivers. My knobby seat and my neck made me realize that in terms of age, I don't exactly belong to the young folks any more.

Despite the bumpy ride, a new sixteen-year-old gang member slumbered in my arms. According to several reports, three people from an enemy gang died at his hands. I hope from the heart that he will soon be able to experience his own Christmas, that through the birth of Christ the spirit of God takes on a form in his life and creates a lasting change. That he is overcome by the peace of God is what I wish for him more than anything in the world, for him and everyone else.

Christmas reminds us Christians of our assignment to be founders of peace. For me, the work for peace and the question of justice belong close together. Henri Nouwen writes in his text, *The Road to Peace,* that Christ will return not as the Christchild, but as a judge, and he will not ask how high are our honors or the influence that we attained, but rather he will ask what we did for the lowest human brother, for strangers, the hungry, the naked, the sick, the imprisoned, the refugee, the slave, the homeless, the crippled, the banished, the ridiculed, the mocked.

Letter from Manila

Philcoa, December 19, 2002. Dear Ones, the story of the three women in Philcoa continues. Marie-Jane, Lane, and Shine have developed in completely different directions.

Marie-Jane, the woman who did not want to share her husband with any other woman, tried to raise her five children alone. For about six months we shared our food with her. For that Marie-Jane helped me in the house and gave me the gift of valuable free time. I hoped that she would find a job before we returned to Switzerland. But then Marie-Jane once again became pregnant—by her "banished" husband! Now and again he did come for a visit to see the children.

Marie-Jane was desperate. In the weeks surrounding the impending birth, her husband decided to return to her entirely. They determined to support his other little family on a regular basis. After the birth of the little boy a few weeks ago, the two were able to be married officially after all these years. The local authorities organized a kind of "mass marriage" on a basketball court for all couples who could not afford a wedding with all of the necessary paperwork. With this unexpected turn, not all of the problems of the eight-person family are solved however. Although the father has a job, his income is so paltry that each unexpected expense could once again cause them distress.

Lane is missing. The court procedures against her husband who raped one of her daughters dragged on for a long time. Many neighbors in the slum and also an aid organization stood at Lane's side. But she began to use those who helped her, borrowed money from her poor neighbors and did not pay it back. She left her young children home alone for days, and no one knew where she had gone. The police are looking for her but today there is no sign of her anywhere.

Shine, with whom I have been reading the Bible for one year, is thankful that her three daughters are healthy and can go to school and that the family lives together peacefully. Her husband, Boy, has unfortunatgely lost his job. In the meantime, Shine has joined a Bible group, and was baptized. Every Saturday she attends "Lilok," a kind of Bible school for slum residents. There she soaks up everything new like a dry sponge. Her husband told her recently that she had changed a great deal for the better. In the meantime, many people come to her house to ask her advice.

Shine, along with some other neighbors, has joined Kamay Krafts, a cooperative for Fair Trade products made by hand, founded by Servants (www.kamay-krafts.org). Now they sew and embroider at home and earn a small but important income. A short time ago, Shine, beaming, made me aware of all that had changed in her neighborhood: the gambling that was going on night and day has stopped entirely. A few addicts of many years' duration have decided to begin a new life, including a few men who inquired about an exchange group of their own. And some of her neighbors have begun to attend the fellowship services of the slum congregation.

Three completely different paths. The good message of God's redemptive love is written in the stories of these three women—and the different human answers thereto.

Warm regards, Christine

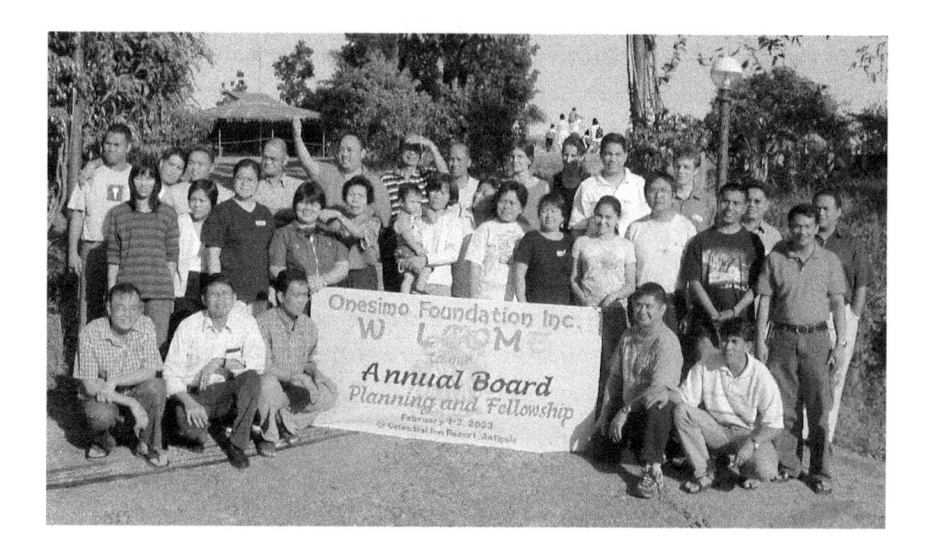

Above, from left to right: Jun Arizala (Pastor), William Docos and Michael Mestiola (two former participants of the Program seven years ago, who now are fully employed), Ezra Martinez (deceased; engineer), Harry Roque (Attorney and University Professor of International Law), David Feliciano (theologian and farmer, Danny Pecio (engineer), Regula Hauser, Christine Schneider, Ruel Billones (psychologist), Daniel Wartenweiler, Dr. Dan Veneracion (dentist), Jerom Turga (attorney).

Middle, from left to right: Baby Gonzales (housewife), Rory Floro (business woman), Pine Gutierrez (Leader of the Philippine Children's Ministries Network (PCMN)), Armi Martinez (social worker), Evelyn Miranda-Feliziano (deceased; theologian and well-known author), Rose Pecio (bookkeeping and administrative director), Ate Grace (manager), Becky Roxas (teacher), Lina Polidario (kindergarten teacher), Hazel Sarol (secretary), BG Polidario (Pastor), Joven Turga (Pastor).

Below, from left to right: Jun Alindogan (teacher and director of the Onesimo-Adult Education), Pepe Gonzales (Pastor), Joshua Palma (youthworker), Manolo Araneta (photographer and agriculturalist), Noel Gabaldon (Pastor, Director, Onesimo).

Life Goes On

In April we will fly "home," to Switzerland. Noel Gabaldon, the overall leader of Onesimo, will move into our little house with his wife, Olen, and his two children. They are looking forward to the little garden, a rarity in the settlements of the poor.

Again and again we speak about Switzerland and how good everything will be. With little success, we try to impart a few ground rules of Swiss culture and etiquette to our two unruly children. A big surprise and help in these attempts is Heidi Berdat. The teacher from Basel arrived in Manila a short time ago for three months and now teaches Noel and Isabel German and arithmetic. That will ease the transfer to Swiss schools. Heidi is a gift from heaven!

I am confident about the future of Onesimo. A crisis in leadership last October gave the Philippine coworkers and our executive committee the necessary signal to keep themselves on the alert, straightforward, and dedicated to the engagement in the concerns of the lost youths we are committed to assist.

Onesimo now consists of five rehab/life-training communities, a school for adult education, leadership training, leisure/camp activities for young people, various self-help projects, guidance for former participants, advocacy for the poor, administration and management of Camp Rock, training of coworkers, and guidance. If possible, our successors will open a new rehab center for girls; all the girls from last July's rehab group are still with us! The Girls' center is now headed, in an honorary position, by Annabel Manalo, a mature woman, psychologist, and teacher at a college. The "Center Mother," our dear Jessica, was able to move into a room at Ingrid and Lothar Weißenborn's little slum house. She already feels like a family member, which alleviates our feelings about departure.

The Weißenborns, a German couple, and also the young Swiss man Daniel Wartenweiler, are in their first language—and culture—year. They would like to join Onesimo.

Last weekend we reached somewhat of a high point before we say farewell here. About thirty of the members of the executive committee, leaders, and honorary coworkers gathered in a two-day retreat on a knoll outside the city. For Christine and me it was very good and motivating to see and feel how enthusiastically the people pray, plan, and share the work and the degree of energy that they muster. The group photo of this meeting will always have a place of honor with us.

According to plan, our airplane is to land in Switzerland on May 1, 2003. After eight-and-a-half years together in the slums, we will move to Basel again. We want to take a month to furnish, settle down, and enroll the children in school. At the beginning of July, I want to begin working at a salaried position, presumably as a professional healthcare provider, and in addition, with all my strength, to be there for Onesimo!

It is now the year 2011. Our family still lives in the same little row house in Basel into which we moved almost eight years ago. Isabel and Noel are now seventeen and fifteen-years-old. For them, our move to Switzerland was not a return but a new beginning.

Their start in school here went extremely well. Both attend the Leonhards Gymnasium in Basel today. But they feel at home nowhere—or perhaps everywhere—and count themselves among the "Third-culture kids." The deep ties that one perhaps develops where one is born and spends one's early years are missing. Although Switzerland is more beautiful, they say, they only feel really well in the tempo, the noise, and the tumult of the people in Manila.

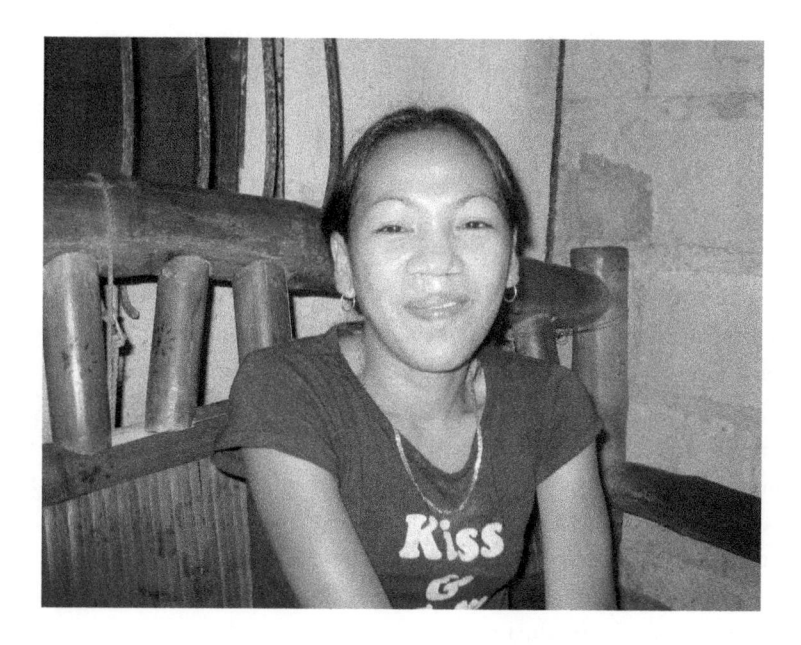

(2007/as a baby, p. 6): I last saw her in 2007, a well-groomed and energetic eighteen-year-old, who still lives with her grandmother and cares for her four younger siblings. In the meantime, Jessabel has finished high school and works as a laundress.

... and what became of them

Since our return to Switzerland, we have flown to Manila regularly. The slums have changed (or not), the people and friends have continued to write their biographies (or have had them written). Here is some additional information about some of the people and places that you encountered in the book.

Manila: Approximately 20 million people live in "Greater Manila," the so-called metropolitan region, today. Air pollution exceeds the toxic emission standards of the World Health Organization three-fold. In the capital region, 7,000 tons of rubbish are deposited daily. In September 2008, the Neue Zürcher Zeitung (a major Swiss daily newspaper) reported that half the population of Manila lives in slums and that 100,000 people from the impoverished provinces join them yearly. Across the country, 44 percent of city residents live in slums. Grotesquely, Manila is the home of the largest shopping center in Asia, the "Mall of Asia," which, among other things, includes an artificial ice skating rink replete with artificial snow.

Bagong Silang (Caloocan City): This resettlement area, my first "home" in the Philippines, has become a suburb. The main streets are jammed to such a degree that I, on my motorcycle, can barely get through. Although I notice individual shops with chic glass fronts, the street seems dirty and dusty, not exactly inviting for a shopping spree. Official tallies number the registered inhabitants at 220,000. Actually, because of the illegal settlers, it is far more. These new arrivals live in newly created slums.

Bagong Barrio (Caloocan City) is still today the densely overbuilt residential area with its wild box-like houses built next to and into one another. A few chic fast food restaurants have been added; the old market was renovated.

Potrero has remained a street slum. The street, in the meantime, has been paved and most of the inhabitants have running water, but the shacks near Araneta Park are more dense than ever. The little Living Spring community that arose at that time continues to try to be a small light in this place. It is animated by the faithful Ate Donita and her women, by Pastor Rico, a handful of happy teenagers and a few individual men.

Navotas: The slum between settlements consisting of houses on stilts and built within a graveyard, is today more densely occupied than seven years ago. One can hardly imagine it if one doesn't see it personally. The preschool run by Ate Juliet was taken over by a British foundation and turned into a grammar school. Now Juliet dreams of a new kindergarten for the large flocks of children in her neighborhood.

Tondo: The well-known Smokey Mountain, from which the scavengers were violently expelled has been demolished in part. The other part constitutes a grass-covered knoll, which one can see from far away. A new rubbish depot, hidden from the street and guarded, empties directly into the ocean. So that the garbage doesn't accumulate to mountain height again, it is regularly loaded onto ships which unload it on a distant island. At the edge of the open garbage dump, a new and terrible slum village is growing. The residential silos newly erected by the government are for the most part occupied by former and active scavengers. Located adjacent to this settlement, one of the ten residential communities of Onesimo continues to operate until this day.

Frisco/Kaingin Bukit: This densely inhabited inner city slum between river bank and factory wall has not changed much. In silhouette, the shacks and houses have become higher by one story because of the newcomers. The Onesimo Community Center was also rebuilt with solid walls and increased by one floor. During the tropical rainstorm with floods in October 2009, approximately sixty people were pulled out of the water that was above the roof terrace. Three children in the neighborhood drowned.

NIA: The incredible thing about NIA is that this slum, since its fire in 1995, has had three more fires. Each time, it has been rebuilt. The endurance of the people is enormous. The little Living Spring Community continues to be led by Pastor B. G. Polidario.

Payatas: After the traumatic rubble collapse, which buried half of the slum village and its inhabitants, the open dump site was closed. But just a short time later, a new mountain of refuse was created immediately adjacent. Finally, in 2009, the old trash heap which had collapsed was again opened as a collection depot. Everything is carefully guarded, to be sure, so that the press can't get in and publish negative headlines. In Payatas, Onesimo opened an additional community with daycare in January 2010.

Philcoa: Following a fire in January 2007, during which the house of the first Girls' Community was destroyed, this slum received a new face. The swamp was dried out and built over, and the last rice fields are gradually disappearing. The houses look more stable since having been rebuilt. The government has built a beautiful multi-use facility on the village plaza. In our former slum house, with the help of the former Swiss ambassador, Dr. Werner Baumann, the third Girls' Center was opened.

Rob and Lorraine Ewing found, after their return to Australia, time and space for processing, rest, and renewal. Both have received further training and have been working for many years as pastors in Western Australia.

Jessabel was the disfigured, undernourished newborn of an addicted teenager, whom I encountered on my first day in Bagong Silang in 1988. Jessabel survived and was operated on at a United States NGO without charge. The last time that I saw her in 2007, she was a well-groomed and energetic eighteen-year-old, who still lived with her grandmother and took care of her four younger siblings. Jessabel has since finished high school and works as a laundress. "I have you to thank for my life," she wrote to me, "and I am very happy with my life!"

Reymond belonged to my bodyguards in 1989, in the "Orphanage" in Bagong Silang. He was fourteen at the time and running from the police. In all these years, I have received mail from him now and again (in which he never asked me for help or begged me for money!). During my last visit to him at home in Bagong Silang in 2007, I experienced him as a loving thirty-three-year-old father of three children. He earns a modest income as the chauffeur of a Jeepney. He and his wife, Bianca, beam at me with open and laughing eyes; even though their one-room corrugated tin house is much too small for their growing family with teenage kids. Both attend the local Christian congregation regularly.

Ana and Rodelio and I did not meet again. I don't know where and how they are living.

Brian, or **Mata** as they called him when he was still "one-eyed," is today a hard-working construction worker who takes good care of his wife and children, so I have been told.

Joel Mangaba is one of the approximately thirty children of our first sponsorship program in Bagong Silang. He early demonstrated an unusual talent for mathematics. Joel worked as director of a technical college in Manila until he was recruited to become a professor at the University of the East. Joel is married to Nivalyn. The childless couple devotes their free time entirely to the Living Spring Community in Bagong Silang. At our last meeting, Joel told me "I am so happy to be able to support Onesimo with a part of my income."

Jovelyn Opiasa, the wife of my first friend and mother of Jonar who suddenly died of dysentery, and I have not seen each other again. One says that she was able to find another husband and lives with him in a province adjacent to Bagong Silang.

Nardo Opiasa has been considered missing for seven years. The meeting in the mountains, where he had withdrawn as a resistance fighter with the NPA, was our last. Presumably Nardo lost his life in a battle with government troops.

Dario Opiasa and Noriel Opiasa, the younger brothers in my first guest family, continue to live in Bagong Silang to this day. Dario is married to Veronica and has a son. Noriel and his wife, Winnie, have four children. Both are responsible fathers and work as foremen at a zoological garden. Dario conscientiously lives according to his evangelical faith, while Noriel is an active member of a Catholic congregation.

James, the trade unionist, is currently forty-five-years-old and works as a security guard. He earns very little, rides to work on his bicycle, and works hard seven days per week. Therefore he doesn't have much chance to attend worship service. Instead, he conducts personal devotions each evening just for himself and listens to Christian radio programs so that he "remains spiritually fit," as he says. James is still single and lives with his aged mother, Aling Epang, in Bagong Silang.

Albert, the teacher, and I have not met again. It is said that he is active in one of the many Christian churches in Bagong Silang.

Nick, the witness, disappeared at that time in the southern part of the city because of fear of reprisal at the hands of the corrupt police. I never heard anything about him subsequently.

Paulo was the first drug addict in Potrero who accepted God and found healing. Like many others, he received credit for a self-help project. And like most of the others, it was not possible for him to pay off his motorcycle taxi completely. He suddenly disappeared for a longer time into the provinces, presumably because he was ashamed. At least he didn't return to his old life as a gangster. Later he took care of his family again.

Papa Dela Cruz remained, until his death a few years ago, a faithful and active member of the congregation in Potrero.

Ate Donita is still today a hardworking woman who enjoys life, who believes in the power of prayer, and is a pillar of the Potrero Living Spring community, that small but still vibrant Christian fellowship in that squatter place.

Jeffry, Ate Donita's son, and his wife, Rosalie, were able to leave their lives as dancers in nightclubs behind. They have five children and are doing well. Jeffry works as a head chef in Dubai.

Ate Gloria sings and preaches still today with much enthusiasm in the small Potrero community. Several of her children are also active there and play guitar in the Living Springs youth group.

Dorie Morden, the beautiful head of several preschools, lives with her husband, a doctor, in the USA.

Jojie Cesista recovered from tuberculosis, married, and became a father three times. The family lived in a province near the city and Jojie worked as a fisherman as part of his wife's extended family. He visited us a number of times in NIA before he died of a recurrence of tuberculosis in 1999.

Edwin, Jojie's nephew who ran away with the cash box of the Potrero community, and I never met again.

Katja, the temporary missionary, today lives with her family in East Switzerland. They are active members of a church congregation.

Christian Auer, who after completion of his dissertation in epidemiology married the beautiful Janice from the Potrero slum, worked several years in various countries in the field of tuberculosis research. At the same time, he helped with Onesimo and Servants projects again and again. In 2008 Christian, Janice, and their two children moved back to Switzerland, where he is there for his frail parents and earns his living with further assignments for the World Health Organization.

Joshua Palma, the activist in the non-violent resistance against the resettlement of the garbage pickers, has been leading the Onesimo community in Tondo for four years now and was co-founder and creative head in the development of Onesimo. He has remained single and works today as a Partner NGO in Servants with the name "Lilok." There he has developed, along with **Regula Hauser**, an alternative eco-farm for training and retreats for slum residents.

Benjie and Emi have survived four firestorms in the NIA slum and have started over again and again. They run a motorcycle taxi and small general store as before.

The "Doña" is still our Camp Rock neighbor. The *Forbes* list of billionaires estimates the fortune of her clan in round numbers for 2005 at 1.3 billion dollars, and for 2007 at 2.6 billion dollars. In the year 2010—after the World Economic Crisis—according to the *Forbes* list, they had to make do with 1.6 billion dollars.

Ron, our foster child from that time, is twenty-seven-years old today, lives with his girlfriend in Payatas and is addicted to gambling. He pursues no contact with Onesimo any longer and lives on his girlfriend's income.

Jessica, who with Christine founded the first Girls' Community, later studied social work and is today one of the important coworkers of Onesimo.

Allen, the former gang leader, fell unhappily in love with the daughter of a pastor. As his love was rejected, he gave up his work as an Onesimo community leader and returned to his previous life. He once again became a garbage picker and took drugs. In the meantime, he appears to be finding his way into a better life with the help of Christians in his neighborhood.

Gerald, the small-time criminal street-kid from Cubao, for whose life we fought for a number of years, lives today with his wife and child in the Frisco slum. His life has been up and down: When things are going well for him, he helps the Onesimo community as a volunteer and takes part in the Lighthouse community. When things are not going well, he returns to his old world, until he catches himself. Fortunately, he is supported by a strong wife.

Jose, the ex-nightclub dancer, as well as his brother, **Antony,** a former street kid, today lead a therapeutic community for boys in Onesimo. Both have completed their high school equivalency, are married, and responsible fathers. **Randy's** squashed foot healed well after the operation. He hardly limped at all thereafter. Randy attended the Onesimoschool and completed the program successfully. He was a well-liked coworker in the communities and the camps. At age nineteen, he returned to his family which lived in the provinces. There he became infected with a dangerous parasite and died in October 2007. His younger brother **Runny,** who also completed a few years of rehabilitation in Onesimo, has supported his parents as a factory worker until this day.

Mylene, the girl who was abused, presently lives in the slum of Payatas with her boyfriend, where she makes ends meet as a vegetable seller. The childless couple appears to be hard working and friendly.

Arol and I ran into each other on my last visit in Payatas. He was sitting in a circle with some men, drinking beer, and called to me: "Hello, Chris, how are you? I am now a good guy!" Whatever he meant by that . . .

Venus and John, the borderline case and the gang leader, have four beautiful and healthy children. They are members in the Onesimo lighthouse Community. Venus appears to be the strong woman in the family. John worked a number of years as an aide in Harry's law office, until he ruined his job situation beyond repair. He goes to the dump site frequently to his old job as a garbage picker to support his family.

Joseph Estrada, the former actor and President of the country who was born in Tondo, was put under house arrest as a VIP prisoner after his arrest in 2001. Doubts regarding the charges of corruption against him as well as the legitimacy of his presidency were raised by his successor Gloria Arroyo. In 2007, Estrada was pardoned by Arroyo. In 2010, he once again was a candidate for the presidency, presenting himself in the campaign as the politician for "Law and Order," but lost to Benito Aquino III (known as Noynoy Aquino).

Marie-Jane was able to struggle along with her children and the husband who had returned to her for a few years in Philcoa and then moved to the province of Laguna nearby. In 2010 we heard that she was well, her husband was working as a family chauffeur, and all her children were attending school.

Shine opened a small pharmacy that is a part of a chain that profitably sells generic medicines in the Philcoa slum in 2006. Whenever we see her, she exudes a joy of life and peace which speak louder than many words.

Hazel Formilleza, in whose parents' home we were able to open the first Onesimo community in 1996, studied psychology and later oversaw the leadership training and youth camps and today belongs to the core of the Onesimo leadership. She is married to Franklyn Sarol and is the mother of a daughter. Franklyn, one of the first Onesimo coworkers, works as a sailor today.

Harry H. Roque, the law student whom I met in October 1989 on the roof of a Jeepney, became a good friend and important supporter of Onesimo. As volunteer president of the executive committee of Onesimo he has decidedly helped us over the years in delicate legal situations. In 2007 a new leadership group took over the responsibility. Among the new members, much to our relief, was Harry's partner in his legal practice, **Joel Butuyan.** As students, both partners, along with others, supported a legal aid effort for the poor, free of charge. To financially reinforce this effort, I was able to turn to the OJC Reichelsheim at that time.

As Onesimo President, Harry and others stepped back in order to remove Onesimo from the line of fire. As a lawyer, high school professor, and political activist, Harry has increasingly become an important "voice of the street" in the country-wide opposition to the corrupt government of Arroyo. Since Gloria Arroyo's accession in 2001, approximately 600 members of the opposition have been murdered or have disappeared without a trace. Even Harry, who fearlessly speaks clearly and objectively on television and radio almost weekly, had repeatedly received death threats. He and his family are prepared, in an emergency, to leave the country immediately. But I believe that he would even be prepared to die in his fight for justice for the poor people of his country.

Pastor Pepe Gonzales is a member of the leadership of Onesimo and teaches at a theological training institute. Until today he is always available if Onesimo or the Potrero community needs his help. His four children have grown up in the meantime.

Rico, the former gangster, even after his turning to Christ, was not a simple character. After a long journey with advances and defeats, he pursued theological training with Pastor Pepe Gonzales. Today Rico is the pastor of the small Christian congregation in Potrero. As I wanted to visit Rico in 2007, I found him severely wounded in the accident ward of the East Avenue Medical Center. He had been attacked and was happy still to be alive. He himself was once like the street kids who had attacked him, he said, "but God has liberated me and given me a new life."

Jesse Sarol, my language teacher in Bagong Barrio and later a co-founder of Onesimo, today lives with his family outside the slums. As the head of a college for sailors and director of a shipping company, he continues to support Onesimo.

Noel Gabaldon, the former overall leader of Onesimo turned over his position during the first leadership crisis after our return to Switzerland to **Armi Martinez.** Armi led Onesimo for a two year period with much diligence and acumen. Noel found various positions and today works as project leader for the Center for Community Transformation (CCT) among the homeless in Manila. He lives with his wife and two children in a residential quarter outside the slums.

Rose Pecio has been the certified bookkeeper of Onesimo since its founding. With her husband Danny and their three children she voluntarily lives in the slum. Rose is the woman who, like no other, experienced and helped bear all the highs and lows of the work with great devotion and persistence up to the present day. She is not only the director of administration, but also, quietly, the heart of the work, and a prudent adviser for the coworkers.

For thousands of children and young people and for many families from the poverty-stricken areas of Manila, **Camp Rock** has become the embodiment of unforgettable vacation experiences. Only the middle class, earning good wages, can usually afford a holiday in such a beach setting. In the stillness of unsullied nature, many have found trust in a benevolent Creator here. Camp Rock has been under constant renovation and expansion. In October 2009 an additional building with guest rooms was dedicated—in the hope that this leisure-time destination can become self-supporting.

Onesimo has survived two crises in leadership since our return to Switzerland. Now the ongoing work can be assured of firm ground (www.Onesimo.ch and for Filipinos: www.Onesimo.ph). This is due, above all, thanks to the Filipino team under the general leadership of **Dennis Manas** and the faithful Philippine executive committee. **Regula Hauser,** our Servants coworker in Manila, responded quickly whenever she was called upon for advice and mediation. **Ingrid and Lothar Weißenborn,** the retired couple from Germany, were also of great help. In past years, they both attended to the ministry of the former Onesimo trainees, the families and single people of the Onesimo Lighthouse Community. Concurrently, they renovated and expanded Camp Rock.

A further milestone for Onesimo was the erection of a training center for a school and professional courses with an auto repair shop. This project was generously supported by the OJC Germany and the leader of Onesimo at that time, Armi Martinez.

The young Swiss man, **Daniel Wartenweiler,** founded a Onesimo branch for very young street children and homeless families. In 2009 he registered this impressive organization under the name "Onesimo Bulilit Foundation" as a separate NGO (www.bulilit.onesimo.ch). Including these Onesimo kids, there are ten Onesimo communities in metropolitan Manila today. Their network of relationships with the urban population, the churches, and NGO's continues to grow. Hundreds of people can get help there every day—and find hope.

Epilogue

We become familiar with them in our easy chairs in front of the television: At least once or twice a year a wave of information rich in images rolls from the Philippines into the climate-controlled living rooms of Central Europe. For a few moments, the rubbish heaps of Manila are shown around the world; the pillar of ash of Pinatubo becomes legendary; the wild-weather coast of the Philippines as a region of record for cyclones and floods is seen as unique.

Known around the world, but far away. Christian and Christine Schneider-Tanner provide a picture that's much more of a close-up. Whoever wades through the slum with them arrives at a lost paradise via a very special school of the senses. One actually smells the pressing need between the lines, hears the scratching of the cockroaches under the bed, and feels the rage in one's own breast in the face of injustice that befalls the people in the slum. But the tour that they lead does not stay on a path limited to the senses; it becomes a journey of the heart. Not only abyss and aversion, but also new messengers of hope consistently reach us through foul odors and twilight: Nick, the chief witness; Jessabel, the doomed; James, the trade unionist; Joshua, the activist; Doña, the billionaire; Allen, the gang leader; Jose, the nightclub dancer; Nardo, the resistance fighter; Mata, the one-eyed; Venus, the borderliner; Harry, the human rights attorney; Arol, the rapist; Bo-Boy, the mass murderer; Albert, the teacher.

Messengers of hope. That's what they are. Because they have no chance and fight nonetheless. Because they seem lost, yet have faith. Because they are weak but love all the same, to the extent that they are able. Because they wander on the narrow ridge between life and death, between rubble and redemption.

These messengers are encouragement and incentive for us. They challenge us to change the table of contents: To see more of our world than the images on the screen transport into our living rooms; to expect more from life than the binding career paths of a self-referential society; to find more to believe in and trust and dare than a cash deposit in an interest-bearing account. Yes, to learn again how to live between rubble and redemption—to make one's own life spacious enough for the unexpected, for the detour, for a life of privation. Only the mendicant is oriented toward angels and miracles.

The change in a table of contents that the book inspires relates not only to the manual of one's own heart. Christian's and Christine's book is also a guide for a new epoch in the shared responsibilities of a global world. Today, protracted aid for development can no longer be a one-way street. Suffering in the world does not first cry out for resolution, but for the ability to empathize, to draw nearer, to experience first hand what is needed. In the two decades as project partners of Onesimo, we in the OJC have received essential inspiration through the work of Christine and Christian for the revision of our world wide undertakings as an NGO: to seek true, transparent partnerships, to strengthen the indigenous roots of initiatives, to encourage self-help and personal responsibility in the locality in order to avoid dependence of all kinds, and in all of this, to leave enough space for the spirit of God, to allow the unexpected to occur.

"God embraces us with reality," the church fathers teach us. Perhaps it is time for one or the other of us to lay aside the remote control and the mouse, and, encouraged by this book, examine one's own heart. One can wait for messengers of hope; one can also attempt to track them down—or to become one oneself. There is much space in our world between rubble and redemption.

Dr. Dominik Klenk
Director and Prior of the Ecumenical Community "Reichelsheim fellowship" (OJC: www.ojc.de).
The OJC has furthered partner projects in developing countries for over three decades.
www.ojc.de/weihnachtsaktion

Acknowledgements

Our thanks go to Willi Näf (www.geistschreiber.ch), who guided us in our writing with enthusiasm and keen expertise. We also received important support for the book from the Gerda and Lukas Ritz family of Bernex, Switzerland, from Ursula and Silvio Albertini of Bubendorf, Switzerland, and from Mrs. Busch, our editor at Brunnen Verlag Gießen.

Regarding the English edition our thanks go to Dagmar Grimm, our excellent translator, to Pieter Kwant of Piquant Editions, to Angela Lewis, Verena Foster, Mylah Roque, and Kristin Jack who were all of great help with the English manuscript.

Moreover, with this book we would like to thank the many people, congregations, and institutions that have accompanied us in some way in the last decade, especially the faithful coworkers in Servants Switzerland. They all are a part of this story, in giving and receiving. Through them countless people in Manila and we ourselves experienced the nearness of God and his care!

Thanks is also due to our partner organizations in Germany: OJC in Reichelsheim (www.ojc.de) and AFEK (www.afek-ev.de): They have been affiliated with the Onesimo Project for many years.

We are also grateful to CVJM/F—Domino Basel, Switzerland, the Federal Ministry for Economic Cooperation and Development (BMZ) in Germany, the German Embassy in Manila, the Governing Council of the city of Basel-Stadt, and the Lottery Funds of the Kanton Basel-Land, Switzerland for the advancement of the infrastructure- and training-projects of Onesimo.

Christian and Christine Schneider

Onesimo is a partner organization of Servants to Asia's Poor and Servants Switzerland (www.onesimo.ch/www.bulilit.onsimo.ch/www.servantsasia.org).

More books from Servants Authors

The Sound of Worlds Colliding edited by Kristin Jack, 2009 Hawaii Printing House, Phnom Penh, Cambodia

The Urban Halo by Craig Greenfield, 2007, Authentic Media, www.authentic-media.co.uk

Servants Among the poor by Jenni M. Craig, 1998, OMF Literature Inc., Metro Manila, Philippines

Companion to the Poor by Viv Grigg, 1984, Albatross Books, 2004 Waynesboro: Authentic and World Vision, 2004

Contact Addresses

Christine and Christian Schneider are available, by arrangement, to speak about the slums and their experiences in English and/or German:

Pilatusstrasse 34, CH-4054 Basel/Switzerland
christian.schneider@onesimo.ch

Contributions

Contributions with the designation "Onesimo" are forwarded directly to Manila to be used for charitable purposes only. Please check with your tax advisor regarding tax deductions.

Postfinance 40-38079-9
IBAN: CH83 0900 0000 4003 8079 9
Payable to: Servants Switzerland 4054 Basel
Purpose: Onesimo

For more information about Servants to Asia's Urban Poor, go to:

www.servantsasia.org
or contact your nearest Servants Office:

Canada	admin.canada@servantsasia.org
United Kingdom	uk@servantsasia.org
United States	usa@servantsasia.org
Australia	Australia@servantsasia.org
New Zealand	nz@servantsasia.org
Philippines	Philippines@servantsasia.org

Cambodia	Cambodia@servantsasia.org
Switzerland	Switzerland@servantsasia.org

Like-minded Groups

A Rocha	www.arocha.org
InnerCHANGE	www.innerchange.org
Servants Partners	www.servatpartners.org
Urban Expression	www.urbanexpression.org.uk
UNOH	www.unoh.org
Urban Vision	www.urbanvision.org.nz
Waiters Union	www.waitersunion.org
Plan B	www.wecan.be
Word Made Flesh	www.wordmadeflesh.com

Lightning Source UK Ltd.
Milton Keynes UK
UKHW010604080819
347613UK00002B/63/P